NAVIGATING SLEEPLESSNESS

A MENTAL HEALTH HANDBOOK

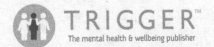

ABOUT THE AUTHOR

Dr Lindsay Browning is a chartered psychologist and associate fellow of the British Psychological Society who runs sleep consultancy and therapy services at her private practice, Trouble Sleeping.

Dr Browning began studying psychology at the University of Leicester, where she obtained a first-class BSc in Psychology. She was then awarded the Wellcome Trust four-year scholarship at the University of Oxford, to study a masters in Neuroscience and a doctorate in Insomnia. During her MSc in Neuroscience, she investigated brain asymmetry in patients with schizophrenia and started to become interested in the field of sleep research. At that time (2002), sleep was still an emerging field of study, where much was not yet understood. Dr Browning's doctoral thesis looked at the relationship between worry, rumination and insomnia.

After graduating in 2006, Dr Browning set up her private practice, Trouble Sleeping, to help people of all ages with their sleeping problems. At that time, there were only a handful of sleep specialists treating insomnia in the UK.

Today, Dr Browning spends her time helping individual clients improve their sleep with cognitive behavioural therapy for insomnia (CBT-I) and also working with companies to offer employee wellbeing programmes. She offers sleep and shift work advice and consultancy to companies and the public sector, including the NHS and the police, as well as charities and other organizations including And So to Bed, to promote healthy sleep and general wellbeing. When she is not working, she enjoys cooking, travel and spending time with her family.

Connect with her online: @DrBrowningSleep
www.troublesleeping.co.uk

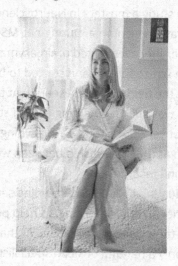

NAVIGATING SLEEPLESSNESS

A MENTAL HEALTH HANDBOOK

HOW TO SLEEP DEEPER AND BETTER FOR LONGER

DR LINDSAY BROWNING

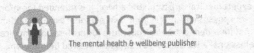

TRIGGER™
The mental health & wellbeing publisher

First published in 2021
This edition published in 2023 by Trigger Publishing
An imprint of Shaw Callaghan Ltd

UK Office
The Stanley Building
7 Pancras Square
Kings Cross
London N1C 4AG

US Office
On Point Executive Center, Inc
3030 N Rocky Point Drive W
Suite 150
Tampa, FL 33607
www.triggerhub.org

A CIP catalogue record for this book is available upon request from
the British Library
ISBN: 978-1-83796-282-2
Ebook ISBN: 978-1-83796-283-9

Typeset by Lapiz Digital Services

ABOUT THIS BOOK

Although the advice offered in *Navigating Sleeplessness* is based on scientific principles for the treatment of sleeping problems, it is designed to be accessible to anyone with no prior knowledge of science. This book attempts to pack a plethora of advice and information into a very short space. The advice is intended for anyone struggling with their sleep, to give them clear and easy-to-implement suggestions for how they can improve it.

This book is intended to be read in order, with subsequent chapters and exercises building on previous chapters. It is laid out so that you will easily be able to refer back to any sections you want to consult in the future. In addition, you will find several "compass points" that highlight especially useful or important information throughout, pointing you in the right direction, as it were.

This book will hopefully empower you to take the steps detailed here to prioritize your own sleep and improve your overall wellbeing. At the end of the book you will find signposts to further resources should you need to seek further professional help for your sleep or mental health.

CONTENTS

Introduction You're not alone 1

Chapter 1 What is "good sleep"? 7

Chapter 2 How much sleep do I need?..................... 25

Chapter 3 What is "bad sleep"?................................. 39

Chapter 4 Changes to help your sleep 79

Chapter 5 Starting to address your sleeping
problems... 105

Where to find help and other resources............... 137

References... 145

INTRODUCTION
YOU'RE NOT ALONE

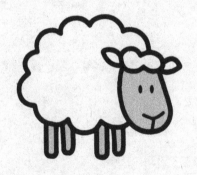

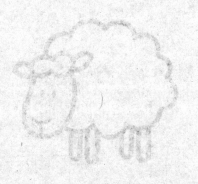

You may be reading this book because you are struggling with your sleep and would like some advice on how to fall asleep faster and stay asleep for longer, or you may be a professional or friend wanting to help someone else with their sleep. This book will offer practical advice on navigating sleeplessness for yourself, or enable you to better help someone else who is struggling with their sleep.

The great thing is that no one is "just a poor sleeper". You can change. This book will walk you through a number of different strategies for overcoming your sleeping problems, and give you techniques to stop your poor sleep from making a reappearance later down the road.

Often, people who struggle to sleep at night feel very alone and desperate. They may have tried giving up caffeine, using over-the-counter sleeping medication, going to bed earlier, going to bed later, using sleep apps and/or trying to improve their sleep hygiene... but nothing has helped. They may find themselves increasingly anxious as bedtime draws near, even having panic attacks at night. They may also spend their days worrying about how their sleep (or lack thereof) is ruining their life.

This book starts with an examination of the science of sleep. This is important because often, people find that they are worrying about an aspect of their sleep that turns out to be perfectly normal and nothing to worry about. We will then move on to explore why sleep is important and how much sleep you should be aiming to get each night. Next, we will examine what can cause your sleep to start to go wrong, including information about a number of potential medical sleep disorders – as well as how stressful life events can disrupt your sleep, causing insomnia. Armed with the knowledge of what your specific sleep issues are, you can start to learn some strategies and techniques to help you fix your sleeping issue. In addition to good sleep hygiene principles, tips for managing nighttime worries and anxieties, this book also provides some relaxation techniques for you to use.

This book should help to give you a clear understanding of why your sleeping problem has developed in the first place and what you can do to stop it. It is a chance to take a good look at your lifestyle and choices to see if there are aspects that are not helping you or are causing you extra stress. You may find that you have developed an issue with sleep due to not taking care of yourself, and this may be an unexpected opportunity – your chance to prioritize your wellbeing. Sleeplessness is a sign that something is wrong in your overall health and wellbeing, and this is your opportunity to fix it.

Whether your sleeping problem has only just started, or you have been suffering with insomnia for many years, read on. I am Dr Lindsay Browning, and I am here to help you navigate sleeplessness.

CHAPTER 1

WHAT IS "GOOD SLEEP"?

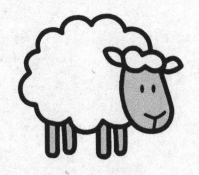

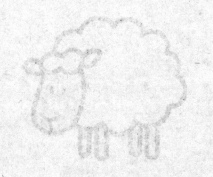

Sleep is arguably *the most important thing* you can do for your body, other than breathing and eating. Before we delve into the specific tips and advice for making sure you are getting enough good-quality sleep, we will first look at what actually happens to your brain and body while you are sleeping.

PLEASE READ THIS CHAPTER FIRST! You may be tempted to skip this science-y part and go straight to the practical advice, but I thoroughly recommend that you read this chapter first. The advice in this book will make a lot more sense once you understand how sleep really works. Also, you would not believe how many people contact me, worrying about their sleep, when it transpires that their sleep is actually completely normal. In fact, some people obsess so much about what they think is their "abnormal" sleep that they actually start to develop a *real* sleeping problem.

So, to start with, let's explore what normal sleep looks like.

THE NATURE OF SLEEP AND WHY IT'S IMPORTANT

Scientists are constantly discovering more and more about what our brains and bodies do while we sleep. Evolutionarily, sleep makes little sense, since it requires you to be unconscious and vulnerable to attack by predators. Sleep must therefore be absolutely vital to our survival to outweigh this risk.

Although you may have experienced pulling an "all-nighter" where you stayed awake for a social or work reason (or because of insomnia), we know that humans cannot survive without any sleep at all in the long term, and regularly getting enough sleep (more on what that means later, but for a healthy adult it would be approximately 7–9 hours) has a great deal of benefits. Generally, studies have shown that getting the right amount of sleep reduces anxiety and depression, and lowers your risk of heart disease, stroke, dementia, obesity, certain hormonal cancers and Type 2 diabetes. It is also correlated with a more robust immune system.

Your brain does not simply "switch off" when you sleep.

So, far from being a period of time when our brains simply "switch off", there are a whole host of incredible processes going on when we sleep. Our brain does this by moving through a series of different kinds of sleep (called sleep stages) in cycles of approximately 90–110 minutes across the night. Each sleep cycle includes light sleep (N1 and N2), deep sleep (N3) and dreaming sleep (R, or REM). As yet, we do not know exactly how each stage of sleep benefits our bodies, but scientists are learning more all the time. Generally speaking, it is thought that deep sleep is where your body physically repairs and regenerates, and it is also where children produce hormones to help them grow. Light sleep may be important for forming long-term memories, and dreaming sleep is where you process emotion and make sense of what has happened that day. You need all stages of sleep to be healthy and happy.

Let's take a look at what these sleep stages look like.

SLEEP STAGES

As you fall asleep, you initially go into the lightest stage of sleep (N1), during which you are very easily woken up – even someone lightly touching your arm or quietly whispering your name will rouse you. During N1, different parts of your brain start to fall asleep, but sometimes they don't all do so at quite the same time. Sometimes, just as you fall asleep, you will experience a jerking sensation that wakes you back up; it may even feel like you're falling. This is known as a hypnic myoclonia (or hypnic jerk), and it is an involuntary muscle spasm that, although frustrating, is perfectly normal, and can more commonly happen if you are stressed or jet-lagged. N1 sleep can last between one and seven minutes at the start of the night.

Next, you go into stage N2 sleep. This is still a light sleep, but you are now not as easy to wake up. In the first sleep cycle, it can last anywhere between 10 and 25 minutes. You will spend most of your night in this stage of sleep overall.

After N2, you will move into a deep, slow-wave sleep – N3. This is where you are so deeply asleep that even a loud noise may not wake you. In the very first sleep cycle of the night, this stage lasts between 20 and 40 minutes.

Sleep Stages

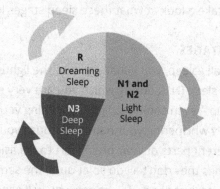

On a side note, children have extremely deep sleep (much deeper than adults), especially in their first sleep cycle, and are very hard to wake during this time. In fact, in a child's first sleep cycle they can be so deeply asleep that they are almost impossible to wake. (This is also why the Tooth Fairy and Santa Claus often choose to visit about an hour after children have fallen asleep!) As we age, we tend to get less and less deep sleep overall, especially men.

After deep sleep comes dreaming sleep (stage R), also known as REM (rapid eye movement) sleep, so named because your eyes will rapidly move underneath your closed eyelids while you are dreaming. (Incidentally, although Freud thought that the content of your dreams said a great deal about your unconscious mind, current scientific opinion does not agree. The only time to be concerned is if you are having repeated nightmares or flashbacks in your dreams that could be related to a traumatic incident – as in post-traumatic stress disorder.)

With the end of dreaming sleep, the first full sleep cycle of the night ends. A brief arousal from sleep may occur before, or at the start of the next sleep cycle. Each full cycle averages around 90–110 minutes, and so a full night's sleep will contain five or six cycles.

In one night, a healthy young adult will spend approximately 23% of the time in dreaming sleep (R), 54% in light sleep (N1 and N2), 18% in deep sleep (N3) and 5% awake.

The graph on the next page shows how these sleep stages change across the night.

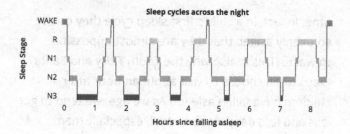

Sleep cycles across the night

As you can see from the graph, as the night progresses, we get less and less deep sleep (N3) and more and more dreaming sleep (R) in each subsequent sleep cycle. As you move down the graph, from being awake through to deep sleep (N3), you move further and further from consciousness and you become harder to wake up. You're closest to consciousness when you're in dreaming sleep (stage R) – in fact, your brain activity while you dream looks very similar to when you are awake. People who say that they "don't dream" almost certainly do; they will just be waking up from a part of the sleep cycle that is not REM sleep (either N2 or N3), so they don't remember their dreams.

People who say that they "don't dream" almost certainly do; they will just be waking up from a part of the sleep cycle that is not REM sleep.

If you wake from REM sleep, not only are you more likely to remember your dreams, but you will also feel relatively alert the moment you wake. This might happen after just one sleep cycle, right at the beginning of the night. You might think, *Wow, that must have been a good-quality 90 minutes sleep, because I feel great!* A 90-minute nap during the day is an ideal length of nap for this reason – because you will likely have completed a full sleep cycle and wake feeling alert. During the night, however, even though you may feel relatively good at that moment, you would soon start to feel sleepy again.

Conversely, if you are woken up from a deeper sleep stage, then you will feel tired, groggy and disorientated when you wake up – what is called "sleep inertia". The further from consciousness you were when you woke (i.e. the deeper the sleep), the greater the inertia, the more your body wants you to go back to sleep.

How you feel the moment you wake up is much more linked to the stage of sleep you are directly woken from, therefore, than the length or quality of your sleep overall. This is worth remembering, because the same is true at the end of the night as at the beginning. For example, have you ever been woken by your alarm at 7am feeling quite refreshed, but then decided to snooze the alarm and lie in? After another half-hour's sleep, you may be confused when you wake up feeling groggier and more sleepy than you did at your original, earlier alarm. You may be cross with yourself and think that you have "ruined" your sleep, or "slept too much". All that happened, however, was that the first time you woke you were in a lighter stage of sleep (nearer consciousness), while the second time your sleep cycle continued into a deeper sleep (further from consciousness). If you wait around 10–15 minutes, your sleep inertia will have passed.

How you feel the moment you wake up is much more linked to the stage of sleep you are directly woken from than the length or quality of your sleep.

"SMART" ALARMS

You can get sleep apps and other technology to monitor your movement through the sleep stages and wake you from an optimal light stage of sleep so that you feel alert immediately upon waking. I am not a huge fan of these "smart" alarms, however, because they do this by waking you at the optimal point *before* you need to wake up, and therefore you may not get as much sleep in total as you would do naturally. Yes, you may wake at 6:15am (from light sleep) feeling more alert than if you woke from deeper sleep at 7am, but you ultimately lose out on 45 minutes of sleep!

I suggest that you wake up with your regular alarm, have something to eat and drink, and then, once your sleep inertia has gone, see how you really feel.

WAKING DURING THE NIGHT

As each sleep cycle ends and sleep moves from dreaming (R) back to light sleep (N1) again, most people will briefly wake up. They may just adjust their covers and roll over. However, people often tend not to remember these periods if the arousal is short. This is because your brain needs to be awake for long enough (at least two minutes) to store the memory of waking up into your long-term memory so you can recall it the next day. Most sleepers wake at least four to five times every night, but they are conscious so briefly that they would swear the next day that they had slept through the night without waking.

Most sleepers wake at least four to five times every night.

When people *do* remember waking up during the night, they may believe that their sleep has been disrupted and is of a poorer quality than if they had "slept through without waking". This is simply not true. As we have seen, sleep is by its very nature already fragmented into sleep cycles. Awakenings are only a problem if you are waking very frequently, for long periods, or the awakenings interrupt your sleep stages (such as you wake up from deep sleep). As we age, these night-time awakenings tend to get longer and more frequent, so we are more likely to remember them the next morning. This doesn't mean we get worse sleep as we get older – merely that we will start to *remember* some of the awakenings we had been having all along!

I see so many people who are worried about the fact that they have been waking up during the night. I try to reassure them that, as long as they get back to sleep relatively quickly and they are only waking a few times in the night, this is part of normal sleep and does not need to be fixed.

Needing the toilet during the night
One more issue that often worries people is needing to go to the toilet during the night – so much so that they often start to significantly limit what they drink in the evening. In reality, needing the toilet is often not the only cause of someone's awakening.

If I were to ask you to think about how often you go to the toilet during the day, you will likely report that you go to the toilet every two to three hours, which is normal. If you have been asleep for two to three hours in the night and you wake up enough to *realize* that you are awake, you will simply become aware of your bladder and find that it is a bit full (in the same way that it would have filled up during the day). The best thing to do is to get up and go to the toilet and then go back to bed. If you radically restrict drinking in the evening, you are likely to wake up in the night simply because you are thirsty!

Obviously, if you drink a very large amount of water right before bed then you will certainly wake bursting to go to the toilet. Instead, try to find a happy middle ground, drinking small amounts in the evening to keep yourself sufficiently hydrated without overloading your bladder. If you are waking numerous times during the night to go to the toilet, or needing to urinate more frequently during the day as well as at night, then you should speak to your doctor to see if something else is going on.

WHEN YOU NEED TO SLEEP AND WHY

Now we know what happens to you while you are asleep, we shall now discuss *when* you sleep. There are two processes in your body that regulate the timing of your sleep: your sleep drive – your body's need for sleep, which increases with time passed since you last slept, and your internal 24-hour clock – also called your circadian rhythm – which tells your body when it's time to sleep. To sleep well and easily, you need to have both a big sleep drive (for which significant time needs to have passed since you last slept) and for it to be the optimal time of day to sleep (which will be at night rather than during the day, for the reasons explained below).

YOUR SLEEP DRIVE

Your sleep drive works in a similar way to hunger: you will feel increasingly hungry as the time passes since you last had something to eat, and then, once you eat, your hunger (your drive for food) will reduce. If you eat a small snack, your hunger will be a little reduced, but not by as much as if you had eaten a full meal. The same thing happens with sleep. The longer it has been since you last slept, the higher your sleep drive and the easier it will be for you to fall asleep. Once you sleep, your sleep drive reduces. The longer you sleep, the more it reduces. If you sleep for a long time, you will greatly reduce your sleep drive, whereas if you only sleep for a few hours or have a short nap, you will only partially reduce your sleep drive. As soon as you wake up, your sleep drive will start increasing once again.

When people are struggling with their sleep, they will often try to grab some extra sleep wherever and whenever they can, believing that getting sleep at any cost is the most important thing.

For example, if you have a terrible night and only sleep for a few hours, your sleep drive will still be very high in the morning, so you may decide to try to get some more sleep rather than getting up at your usual wake time. You may even call in sick for work or postpone your morning plans so that you can have a lie-in. This may give you a few more hours' sleep, but it also means that you have now significantly reduced your sleep drive. If you had got up at the usual time and powered through the day on *less* sleep, your sleep drive would have been higher throughout the day (not fun, I know) but you would find getting to sleep much easier that night. The same thing happens when you have a nap to make up for a poor night's sleep. The afternoon nap will refresh you, but it will also make it harder for you to fall asleep that evening (due to the reduced sleep drive).

Don't allow yourself to compensate for a bad night's sleep.

It might seem paradoxical, but if you don't allow yourself to compensate for a bad night's sleep, then sleep the following night will be easier (due to your having a higher sleep drive). This way you can start to break your ongoing pattern of night after night of poor sleep.

YOUR INTERNAL CLOCK

Another important factor that controls your alertness and sleepiness across the day and night is your internal 24-hour clock, otherwise known as your circadian rhythm. You probably won't ever be aware of it unless you travel across many time zones and suddenly you're faced with the strange experience whereby your body is telling you it is time to go to bed when the country you're in is just waking up.

Your circadian rhythm is how your body knows what time it is without needing to look at a watch, and why you feel alert and awake during the daytime and sleepy at night. In addition to telling your body when to sleep and wake, it directs your cardiovascular system, drives your metabolism and determines when your body repairs cells and fights infections. It also dictates when your body best digests food and when it produces hormones.

One of these hormones is melatonin, which tells your body that it is the right time to sleep. Thus, with jet lag, you may be very tired when it is nighttime and *want* to sleep (your sleep drive may be high because you have been awake for a long time), but if your body has not produced melatonin because your body's circadian rhythm thinks it is still daytime, then you will find it hard to sleep, despite your high sleep drive.

Light exposure helps to establish our circadian rhythm. Our eyes not only send signals to our brain's visual cortex so that we can see images – they are also directly connected to the suprachiasmatic nucleus (SCN), which controls our circadian rhythm. Bright light exposure lets our brain know that it is daytime, while dim or no light exposure tells us it's night. Problems with our circadian rhythm can therefore occur when people work night shifts and don't get bright light exposure at the right times of day. In addition, some people who are blind can find that their circadian rhythm is not set to a regular 24-hour rhythm, as their eyes are not able to pass the necessary information to the SCN.

Bright light exposure lets our brain know that it is daytime, while dim or no light exposure tells us it's night.

We also have a natural dip in our alertness just after lunch, when our bodies instinctively want us to have an afternoon nap or siesta. There are many countries, especially in hotter climates in mainland Europe, where a siesta is (or at least was) the norm. In these places, shops and business shut for a few hours at lunchtime to give people time for a long lunch and then a nap. As well as avoiding the hottest part of the day, this afternoon nap allows people to empty their sleep drive a little, helping them to feel refreshed and more awake for the remainder of the day.

You may remember that in the section above I recommend that you try *not* to nap if you are struggling to sleep at night – and this is very true. However, if you are not struggling with your sleep at night, then there is no reason not to take an afternoon nap. Indeed, there are studies to suggest that an intentional powernap of up to 20 minutes would be an excellent way to increase productivity in business. The reason that a nap should not be much longer than this is because we don't want to go from light sleep (stages N1 and N2) into deep sleep (stage N3), or else (as discussed on page 15) we will wake up from the nap feeling groggy. If you can take a 90-minute nap and have a full sleep cycle, then that is even better – though you will have to have a very understanding boss indeed!

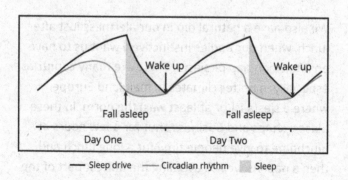

Wake up

Wake up

Fall asleep

Fall asleep

Day One

Day Two

— Sleep drive   — Circadian rhythm   ▓ Sleep

CHAPTER 2

HOW MUCH SLEEP DO I NEED?

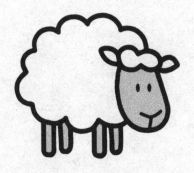

With an understanding of what "good" sleep should look like, let's now find out if you're getting enough of it and why that's important.

NATIONAL SLEEP FOUNDATION RECOMMENDATIONS

The National Sleep Foundation (Hirshkowitz et al., 2015) produced a guide to the recommended amount of sleep people should be getting over their lifetime.

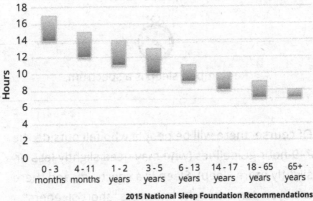

2015 National Sleep Foundation Recommendations

As you can see, as people age their need for sleep decreases. Babies sleep for most of the day, and then as they grow they tend to need less and less sleep toward adulthood. Even as adults our need for sleep changes over time, with older adults (those reaching retirement age) often needing less sleep than they did when they were younger. The chart above is a good guide to what your overall sleep needs are over a 24-hour period – and don't forget that naps count toward your sleep total. Often retirees have more opportunity to nap than their working-age counterparts, and also potentially need less sleep overall. This can result in older people believing that they are not sleeping well enough. For example, they may not sleep for seven hours at night, but may have had plenty of sleep during the overall 24-hour period if you include naps.

Remember: sleep is a spectrum.

Of course, there will be people who fall outside the 7–9-hour guidelines (who may need slightly less or slightly more sleep). Sleep is a spectrum, and there are even some people, known as "short-sleepers", who have a rare genetic variation casing them to need significantly less sleep than the average person (only 4–6 hours, rather than 7–9) to feel fully rested (Shi et al., 2019). Think of the graph above only as a way to see if you are in approximately the right zone. If you feel well-rested during the day, then it is likely that you are getting enough sleep to fulfil your individual sleep needs. Only if you are significantly outside the guidelines might you want to take a moment to think about whether you are getting the right amount of sleep and why.

It is important to remember that there is no need to try to fix something that isn't broken. Striving to deliberately change your sleep so that you can fit into the 7–9 hour guidelines for a working-age adult is not helpful if you are giving yourself sufficient opportunity to sleep and feeling refreshed during the day. There are plenty of people who only sleep for 6 hours per night, for example, and show no negative effects in their daytime functioning.

If it isn't broken, don't try to fix it! Don't force yourself into the sleep recommended guidelines if you feel fine during the day.

There is no perfect number when it comes to the hours of sleep you should be getting each night, although, as we have already mentioned, there is a lot of scientific evidence to suggest that somewhere between seven and nine hours per night is the "Goldilocks zone" where you reap the most health benefits from sleep. If you are consistently getting much more or much less than that, then this may start to affect your health and wellbeing. It is also worth noting that the link between getting too little or too much sleep and health problems is not always causal. For example, sometimes people may be getting much longer than nine hours' or much less than seven hours' sleep because they are sick, rather than their sleep causing the illness.

Scientific evidence suggests that somewhere between seven and nine hours per night is the "Goldilocks zone" where you reap the most health benefits from sleep.

What is definitely *not* conducive to health, however, is to stress or be overly concerned about getting the exact recommended number of hours of sleep, as there is huge variation in people's sleep needs.

To find out if you are getting the right amount of sleep for *you*, answer the questionnaire on the page opposite.

Questionnaire – Getting enough sleep?

First, let's look at how much sleep you are actually getting.

Think about the past week (or the past month if your last week has been unusual).

On average, how much sleep do you get at night during the week?

_____ hours _____ minutes

Do you get a different amount of sleep at the weekend? (Yes/No)

If so, how much sleep do you get at the weekend?

_____ hours _____ minutes

Do you take any naps? (Yes/No)

If so, how many days per week do you nap?

_____

On average, how long do you nap for?

_____ hours _____ minutes

Take a look at your sleep numbers above and compare them to the recommendations for your age (see page 27). If you regularly nap, or sleep for much longer at the weekend, take that into account. As we've seen, if you average 6 hours' sleep each night but you also regularly have a 90-minute nap in the afternoon, this would be an average of 7 and a half hours' sleep in total each day.

If you are getting the right amount of sleep but still feeling tired or sleepy during the day, then this may be a sign of another underlying medical issue. Make sure you speak to your doctor about this and take a look at the section "Other sleep disorders" on page 54.

If you are not getting the recommended amount of sleep per night, then there may be two reasons for this. Either you are not getting enough sleep because you are not prioritizing your sleep, or you're struggling to get to sleep or stay asleep even though you have given yourself the opportunity to do so. When you struggle initiating sleep, maintaining sleep, waking too early or have non-restorative sleep, this is indicative of a sleep disorder (see page 54). This is very different to people who struggle to get sufficient sleep due to their lifestyle.

THE IMPORTANCE OF PRIORITIZING YOUR SLEEP

Not that long ago, CEOs and successful world leaders were suggesting that the key to success was getting as little sleep as possible, promoting the benefits of training yourself to sleep less so that you can have more hours in the day to be successful. For example, Donald Trump, in his book *Trump: Think Like a Billionaire: Everything You Need to Know About Success, Real Estate, and Life* (Trump & McIver, 2004), wrote that he only gets around four hours' sleep per night, and encouraged people to follow his example: "Don't sleep any more than you have to. I usually sleep about four hours per night... How can you compete against people like me if I only sleep four hours?"

However, we now know the long-term damage that can be done by curtailing your sleep, and that not sleeping enough is associated with an increased risk of cancer, Alzheimer's disease and obesity, to mention but a few issues. Margaret Thatcher and Ronald Regan both famously got by on very little sleep, and both of them suffered from Alzheimer's disease at the end of their lives. Now, we cannot categorically say that their lack of sleep caused Alzheimer's, but there is growing evidence to suggest that it certainly did not help. A recent neuroimaging study (Fultz et al., 2019) has shown exactly how the sleeping brain is physically washed clean of amyloid plaques during non-REM sleep. Amyloid plaques are the sticky substances that clog up the brain and are a cause of Alzheimer's. This is just one example of how your body regenerates and repairs itself as you sleep, and it is thought that if you don't get enough of the right kinds of sleep, then your body will simply not have enough time to carry out these necessary processes that keep you healthy.

If you are not getting as much sleep as you need because you are too busy with work or family, and you are regularly putting other things first, then I would encourage you to take a look at your life and consider taking care of *you* first. It is not selfish to prioritize looking after yourself, because in the end you will be better able to look after everyone else if you are healthier and have more energy.

It is not selfish to prioritize looking after yourself.

Remember, if you intend to go to bed at a certain time, try to get rid of things that will interfere with this, like phones, TV and that last-minute email check before bed.

SLEEP AND WEIGHT GAIN

Studies show that people who do not get enough sleep put on more weight than those getting 7–9 hours per night. I hear so many people talk about how they set their alarm an hour or two earlier in the mornings so that they can fit in a gym session before work. Unfortunately, sacrificing sleep to exercise is simply robbing Peter to pay Paul! All your good work at the gym will be undone by the damage done to your health and likelihood of weight gain linked to not sleeping enough. In one study (Xiao et al., 2013), people who reported less than five hours' sleep a night were found to have a 40% higher risk of developing obesity compared to those getting 7-8 hours. In fact, people who don't get enough sleep tend to eat an extra 300 calories per day on average, especially in foods that are fatty or processed. The reason for this is that lack of sleep affects the two hormones that regulate hunger: leptin and ghrelin. When we don't get enough sleep, we don't produce enough leptin, which helps us to feel full, and so we tend to eat more before we feel satisfied. We also produce too much of the hormone ghrelin, which makes us feel even hungrier than usual.

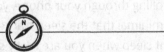

People who don't get enough sleep tend to eat an extra 300 calories per day on average.

SLEEP TRACKERS

Sleep trackers are increasingly popular with people who are interested in their sleep. They are often an included feature of many commonly worn smart watches, or an app you can download to your phone, making them very easy to use. However, I rarely recommend that my patients use a sleep tracker when trying to resolve their sleeping issue. Obviously, technology will continually evolve and improve, but at the time of writing I find that the data is not as accurate as you might want or expect in order to be helpful.

For example, many wearable sleep trackers or apps that require your phone to be placed on your bed or under your pillow use movement data to try to sense when people are sleeping or awake. However, many people with a sleeping problem will lie in bed perfectly still for hours as they try to sleep because they do not want to move and "wake themselves up". This means that their sleep tracker might think that they were asleep when they were not. Also, if you are lying in bed scrolling through your phone, your movement will be so minimal that the sleep tracker may think you are in light sleep when you are really still awake.

Some of the most recent sleep trackers are beginning to use ECG (electrocardiogram) data to include heart rate monitoring as part of the sleep algorithm, which is an improvement, but at present, polysomnography (PSG), which measures brain EEG during sleep to record and analyze the different brain waves produced in the different stages of sleep, is considered the gold standard.

Another issue with sleep trackers is the phenomenon of "orthosomnia", the quest for perfect sleep, which paradoxically often results in worse sleep! People may become so concerned with improving their sleep that they actually start to sleep worse than they did before. I often hear from people who started using a sleep tracking device and, after seeing their sleep data, erroneously concluded that they had a sleeping problem. For example, they may see from the data that they are waking up four or five times during the night and conclude that their sleep is "broken", when in fact, as we have seen, this is completely normal. Another common worry is that their tracker shows that they're "only" spending, say, 25% of their night in deep sleep. Again, this is completely normal. As we have learned, deep sleep does not equate to good sleep, because we need all the different types of sleep (N1, N2, N3 and R) to give us all the benefits of sleep. If 100% of your night consisted of deep sleep, then you would not be healthy. Also, we get less deep sleep as we age, so just because you got nearly 20% deep sleep when you were 25 years old does not mean you will still get that much deep sleep at 60. Remember: if it isn't broken, don't try to fix it!

"Orthosomnia", the quest for perfect sleep, paradoxically often results in worse sleep!

Having said that, there are a few situations in which sleep trackers can be useful. Occasionally they can highlight an issue of which the user was previously unaware. Numerous awakenings during the night could be a sign of sleep apnoea (see page 58), while restless sleep with lots of movement could be an indication of periodic limb movement disorder (see page 63). Also, sleep trackers can be used to help people with paradoxical insomnia (page 56) to realize that they are getting more sleep than they think they are.

CHAPTER 3

WHAT IS "BAD SLEEP"?

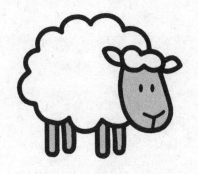

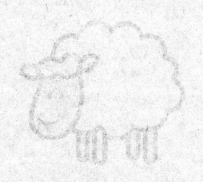

Now that we've seen what healthy sleep looks like, ask yourself: have you been worrying about something that turns out to be a normal part of sleep? If the answer is yes, then great! If, however, after assessing your sleep following the guidelines in Chapter 2, you still believe there is a problem with your sleep, then this chapter will help you identify it.

If you are struggling with your sleep or your energy levels throughout the day, there are a number of potential reasons for this. You could have temporary bad sleep (caused, for example, by a current stressful situation or another factor such as a new baby stopping you from sleeping well right now); you may have a longer-term problem with getting to or staying asleep (a type of insomnia) without a known cause; or you could have another medical sleep disorder. These types of potential causes of sleeping problems are discussed in detail below.

Remember that daytime fatigue can also be caused by a non-sleep-related problem, such as a thyroid issue, anemia, or a viral infection, to name but a few. In addition to these physical issues, mental health issues such as major depression, anxiety and post-traumatic stress disorder (PTSD) can also cause daytime fatigue and sleep disturbances. If your sleeping problem is primarily caused by a factor other than a sleep-specific issue, then it is important to seek help from your doctor to find out what could be causing it and to get tailored help. The advice and tips in this book will only be effective for issues where an inability to fall asleep or stay asleep is not caused by another medical or clinical mental health issue.

HOW DOES TEMPORARY BAD SLEEP DIFFER FROM INSOMNIA?

When people go through a stressful life event, such as a bereavement, relationship breakdown or significant job stress, their sleep will be affected. Even a very good sleeper will struggle to fall asleep or may wake in the early hours with their mind racing at times like this. Other things that can affect your sleep in the short term are jet lag or an unexpected period of broken sleep – due to looking after a sick child during the night, for example.

Each of these understandable disruptions to your sleep should start to have less and less impact as time goes by. For example, the initial grief of a bereavement will eventually become more bearable (though no less sad); you may move on from your negative relationship and either start to feel happy living alone or find love with a new partner; and that stressful time at work will soon pass. However, what often happens is that what should have been a temporary sleeping problem caused by the initial stress or sleep disruption continues long after the cause or "trigger" has gone.

The main reason people may find that they are still sleeping poorly when the trigger is no longer there is, paradoxically, precisely because they start to worry about their lack of sleep. They may become anxious about how little they have slept and change their behaviour when it comes to sleep. This unhealthy focus on sleep and sleeplessness causes the sleep problem to get worse and worse and to take on a life of its own.

An unhealthy focus on sleep and sleeplessness causes sleep problems to get worse.

The difference between a good sleeper and a poor sleeper is that a good sleeper passes through the temporary sleep blip and their sleep recovers once the trigger goes away, while the poor sleeper may start to react to their transitory poor sleep, focusing all their attention on it until it becomes a longer-term, more serious issue. In Chapter 5 we will look at some ways that you can reduce worry about your poor sleep and manage these anxious thoughts.

HOW A TEMPORARY SLEEPING PROBLEM BECOMES A LONG-TERM ISSUE

As we have touched on, when you sleep poorly, you may start to worry about your lack of sleep and how it will affect your ability to function in the daytime. You may start to change your routine and/or behaviour in an attempt to ensure that you sleep better, by going to bed earlier in the evening, for example, or avoiding late-night socializing. You may start to have a nap in the afternoons to catch up on the sleep that you're not getting at night, or even call in sick for work (or quit work altogether).

Every one of these actions is extremely damaging to your sleep and will in fact likely cause the sleep problem to continue for much longer than it would have done otherwise.

The more time you spend in bed *trying* to sleep, the more time you will spend in bed being anxious and not sleeping. Then not sleeping in bed becomes a habit, and you start to fear going to bed, since you expect not to sleep well. Your increased thoughts about sleep during the day and night will lead to higher levels of anxiety and worry about sleep throughout the day, making sleep even harder at night.

The more time you spend in bed trying to sleep, the more time you will spend in bed being anxious and not sleeping.

Think back to when you were sleeping better. Did you do anything to get to sleep? Of course not! Good sleepers do nothing to help them sleep; they simply lie in bed, close their eyes and sleep happens. The problem is, when you start to sleep poorly, you naturally try to fix the problem. After all, it's what we do when we face other issues in life. If you have a problem at work, for example, then you might put in longer hours or learn new skills. If you wanted to be a better golfer, you would practice more and perhaps get some golf lessons.

Good sleepers do nothing to help them sleep; they simply lie in bed, close their eyes and sleep happens.

Sleep, however, is the one thing in life you cannot do better at by trying harder. In fact, it is the opposite – the more you try to sleep better, the worse your sleep will get. This is how a temporary sleeping problem can morph into a longer-term issue. All of the behaviours, thoughts and actions you have initiated in an attempt to fix your sleeping problem have paradoxically made the sleeping problem much worse. Even when the initial cause of your temporary sleeping problem is resolved, these thoughts and anxieties about sleep and the changes you have made to your behaviour will still be there, and they will only serve to perpetuate your sleeping problem.

Sleep is the one thing in life you cannot do better at by trying harder.

THE ORIGIN OF YOUR SLEEP PROBLEM

Think about your sleeping problem. Can you remember if there was a specific event or set of circumstances that occurred back when it first started? It could be something as simple as a bad experience of jet lag, or maybe you were going through a particularly stressful time at work. For many people, the start of the coronavirus crisis in early 2020 triggered a period of poor sleep, due to the worry and stress experienced at that time.

If you are sleeping poorly and you are currently experiencing a stressful or emotional event, then remember that it is understandable that your sleep will be affected. You can use some of the general advice in this book to help minimize the sleep disruption you are facing, but remember that your bout of bad sleep should pass once the stressful time has passed, or at least dissipated.

If your sleeping problem has persisted long since the trigger has disappeared, however, then you will need to change some of the thoughts and behaviours surrounding sleep itself that will have likely developed since, as these will be perpetuating the problem.

Sometimes we do not stop to understand how a sleeping problem has developed. It can be helpful to think about it. Write down how your sleeping problem started (if you can remember a trigger) and how it has changed over time.

HOW DOES STRESS AFFECT YOUR SLEEP?

The tiger in your bedroom

Here is my favourite analogy to explain how stress and anxiety affect sleep.

Imagine that you are snuggled up in bed with your favourite pillows, with bed linen that has been freshly laundered. The room is dark and quiet and you have had a long, successful, busy day. You don't have any worries and you feel as relaxed as can be, content and calm. You are physically tired and ready for a good sleep. You gently start to close your eyes. Just as you are about to drift off to sleep, there is a noise, and suddenly a tiger comes into your bedroom. There is a real-life, three-metre-long adult tiger at the foot of your bed.

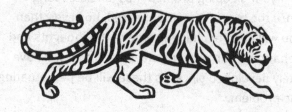

How do you feel?

I bet that, no matter how calm and sleepy you were feeling five seconds ago, you are now feeling incredibly panicked and anxious. Your heart will be racing. Your breathing will be fast and shallow. There is no way in the world that you could possibly fall asleep right now. In fact, if that tiger stayed in your room for ten minutes, one hour, three hours or even all night, you would not fall asleep for a second. No matter how sleepy you had just been feeling, you would be completely unable to fall asleep with a tiger in your bedroom.

This analogy may sound fanciful, but it is a fantastic example of how anxiety stops us from sleeping.

Ever since our caveman days, our bodies have been biologically designed to react to stressful or threatening situations in a certain way – namely, by increasing our adrenaline and cortisol levels, making our heart beat faster and quickening our breathing.

This is what's called our "fight or flight mechanism" at work. When we encounter a physical threat, such as a tiger, we either need to fight it or run away from it in order to survive. By helping you pump more oxygen around your body quickly, this evolutionary mechanism makes either option – an epic showdown or a hasty retreat – easier.

Now, you may be thinking, *But what has this got to do with my sleep? I don't have trouble sleeping because there is a tiger in my bedroom – it's not as if my life is ever in danger when I'm tucked up in bed!*

Granted, in life, we rarely face life-or-death situations such as the tiger in our bedroom scenario. Instead, the "threats" we face from day to day are those of redundancy or serious health scares, and these cannot be fixed by fighting or running away. Nevertheless, our fight-or-flight mechanism kicks in regardless. When you are anxious about the fact that you are not sleeping, your body interprets your potential lack of sleep as a threat and responds in the most basic way it knows how. In order to sleep well, therefore, we need to stop being anxious about not sleeping.

In order to sleep well, we need to stop being anxious about not sleeping.

Stress, worry and sleep

You have likely experienced a poor night's sleep right before an important exam or a critical business presentation, when you really need to be at your best. This happens because when you are stressed, anxious or worried about something, your cortisol levels increase. As discussed on the previous page, cortisol, a hormone produced in your adrenal gland, is part of your fight-or-flight mechanism. It affects the body in a number of ways, giving you more energy, regulating your blood pressure and increasing your blood sugar level. It also has a role to play in your sleep/wake cycle. As we saw with the tiger in your bedroom analogy above, increased cortisol will make it much harder to fall asleep.

In addition to the physiological effects of stress on the body, it also affects your mental processing. If there is something worrying or stressful on your mind, you are likely to ruminate on the problem at night. In today's busy world, when everyone is too busy during the day with work, families, friends and chores, there is often very little time to stop and think. When you lie down in bed at night, it might be the first moment of the day that you have had to reflect on what is really on your mind or in your heart. This is when you might find your mind racing with all the worries and thoughts you hadn't had time to ruminate on during the day. They rush in all at once and they are so loud and busy that you can't get to sleep.

When you lie down in bed at night, it might be the first moment of the day that you have had to reflect on what is really on your mind or in your heart.

Sleep will be easier when the stress and worry reduce, if you make time to deal with your thoughts and anxieties during the day, or if you use some relaxation techniques to help calm your mind at bedtime. (We will discuss some relaxation techniques on page 124.)

Hypervigilance

When you are struggling to sleep, and then you start to worry about the fact that you are not sleeping well, your brain becomes hypervigilant to threats that may disrupt sleep. What this means is that you will start to listen extra hard for any noises that you fear may wake you up. You might find that you are suddenly extra sensitive to sounds – such as a dripping tap two houses away! If you were sleeping normally, you wouldn't be actively listening for such noises and therefore wouldn't notice them. As soon as you are focused on your sleep, however, you start to see everything as a potential threat to your sleep. You may suddenly find your bed partner's breathing very annoying, thinking it is too loud and disruptive and that it is preventing you from sleeping. You might find yourself wanting to sleep in a different room to them, even though you have previously shared a bed for years without issue.

As soon as you are focused on your sleep, you start to see everything as a potential threat to your sleep.

As well as being hypervigilant about external noises, you may also start to notice your own body more. You might find yourself listening to your own heartbeat or becoming very aware of your own breathing, wondering whether it is too fast and preventing you from sleeping. You might also monitor yourself for signs that you are falling asleep. As mentioned in Chapter 1, in the earliest part of sleep, N1, you may experience what's known as a hypnic jerk. This occurs as your muscles start to relax with the onset of sleep, but something wakes you up, at which point they immediately become tense, which results in a sudden jerking or falling sensation. This is very likely to happen if, as you were falling asleep, your brain was trying to *sense* whether your body was falling asleep. Paradoxically, the very act of "seeing if you were about to fall asleep" has actually prevented you from sleeping, and this vicious cycle can repeat itself many times through the night.

SPECIFIC SLEEPING PROBLEMS

We will now look in detail at several specific sleeping problems, beginning with insomnia. We will cover:

- Chronic insomnia
- Paradoxical insomnia
- Obstructive sleep apnoea (OSA)
- Teeth grinding
- Periodic limb movement disorder (PLMD)
- Restless leg syndrome (RLS)
- Narcolepsy
- Sleep paralysis
- Night terrors
- Sleepwalking
- Circadian rhythm disorder (CRD)

CHRONIC INSOMNIA VS SHORT-TERM INSOMNIA

As we have already discussed, short-term sleeping problems, often with an identifiable cause, are common. However, when the sleeping problem, not fully explained by a mental health issue, medical problem or other sleep disorder, continues for a longer time (often due to our reactions to the sleeping problem itself), insomnia can develop.

To be classified as insomnia, the sleeping problem will have an effect on your daytime functioning and also cause difficulties with initiating and/or maintaining sleep at night. It might also cause you to wake up too early. If you are not getting sufficient sleep because you are not allowing yourself sufficient *time* to sleep (e.g. you go to bed at 1am and get up at 6am), then this is not insomnia; it is a lifestyle choice causing a lack of sleep. Nor is the sleeping problem classified as insomnia if it is caused by a mental health condition (such as post-traumatic stress) or other medical/sleep issue.

Clinical diagnosis for insomnia separates the issue in terms of duration. It is classed as short-term (also known as acute) insomnia if the problem has occurred for fewer than three months, whereas chronic insomnia is a sleeping problem that has been going on for longer than this. CBT-I, cognitive behavioural therapy for insomnia, is the recommended treatment of choice for chronic insomnia (see pages 140-141 for information on where to find access to CBT-I), but other changes to one's general sleep hygiene can be effective for shorter-term sleeping issues.

Is it insomnia?

Think about the past week (or the past month if this week has been unusual). On at least three of the seven nights, have you:

1. Taken longer than 30 minutes to fall asleep?
2. Woken up in the night and spent longer than 30 minutes awake before you fell back to sleep again?
3. Woken up more than 30 minutes earlier than your ideal waking time (e.g. before your alarm clock)?
4. Woken up in the morning feeling unrefreshed?
5. Felt that your sleeping problem caused daytime impairments to your mood or ability to function?
6. Given yourself sufficient opportunity to sleep?

If you answered yes to question 1, this is a problem with **initiating sleep**, called **initial insomnia**.

If you answered yes to question 2, this is a problem with **maintaining sleep**, called **middle insomnia**.

If you answered yes to question 3, this is a problem with **waking too early**, called **late insomnia**.

If you answered yes to question 4, this is a problem with **non-restorative sleep.**

If these sleep issues (questions 1, 2 or 3) have been ongoing **for three months or more**, and you also answered yes to questions 5 and 6, then you may meet the clinical criteria for **chronic insomnia**.

If these sleep issues (questions 1, 2 or 3) have been ongoing **for less than three months**, and you also answered yes to questions 5 and 6, then you may meet the clinical criteria for **short-term insomnia**.

Remember: in either case your sleep problem must not be better explained by another medical, sleep or mental health issue.

If you only answered yes to question 4, then your sleep issue may be entirely explained by a different sleep disorder, see "Other sleep disorders", below.

Alternatively, you may have more than one of these sleep issues (e.g. a problem **initiating sleep** and also with **non-restorative sleep**).

PARADOXICAL INSOMNIA

It is important to highlight a subtype of insomnia (not mutually exclusive of initial, middle and late insomnia) called **paradoxical insomnia**. This is when people believe that they have not slept at all the whole night (despite trying to), perhaps for several days in a row, while scientific measurement of their sleep would suggest that they were in fact asleep. People with paradoxical insomnia may also report sleeping very few hours per night, such as only averaging three hours of sleep each night. At present, there is not enough scientific research on this relatively rare sleep problem, but it would appear that people with paradoxical insomnia maintain some ability to monitor their external environment even while sleeping – giving them the impression that they did not sleep at all, or for a very short amount of time. Typical CBT-I (the gold standard treatment for insomnia) will not be appropriate for people with paradoxical insomnia, so if you suspect that this may be your sleeping issue, it is important to speak to your doctor, who may wish to refer you to a sleep clinic for an overnight sleep assessment.

Other sleep disorders

There are a number of other reasons that people may find it difficult to sleep. The sleep disorders described below can occur alone or with insomnia. To help you identify whether you may have one of these sleep disorders, answer the questions associated with each one, with a bed partner if you have one, as some are about what you do when you are asleep, and you may not be aware of the symptoms happening at the time.

OBSTRUCTIVE SLEEP APNOEA (OSA)

- Do you snore?
- Do you wake during the night gasping for breath?
- Has your partner noticed that you stop breathing in the night?
- Do you sometimes wake up from dreaming that you are choking?
- Do you sleep for the right amount of time, but still feel exhausted during the day?
- Do you wake with a headache in the morning?

If you answered yes to any (or several) of these, you may have **obstructive sleep apnoea** (OSA).

OSA is a sleep disorder that causes you to stop breathing during the night, often as a result of a blockage in your airway. Your muscle tone is reduced at night, making it more likely for your throat and tongue to press against your airway. If there is a blockage in your airway (such as if your throat has closed up or your tongue is blocking the back of your throat), then you will not be able to get fresh oxygen into your lungs, and there will start to be less and less oxygen circulating in your blood. When you have not breathed for a while, the oxygen content in your blood will get to a low enough level to signal a problem, and your body and brain will actively wake you up to get you to start breathing again. This awakening will often be accompanied by a big gasp of breath. These awakenings can happen hundreds of times per night, but you will most likely not remember many (or any) of them, as you will fall back to sleep almost immediately afterwards.

Regardless of whether you remember it or not, however, if you are being woken repeatedly in the night, then your sleep cycles will not be the continuous waves as shown in the graphs earlier in the book. As we have already discussed, waking briefly between each sleep cycle is normal (between R and N1); waking repeatedly within the stages themselves (N1, N2, N3 and R) is not. Without consolidated sleep, you will not get the necessary benefits from any sleep you do get. With OSA, people wake up after having what they thought was 7–9 hours of good-quality sleep still feeling exhausted (because, unbeknownst to them, they have not really slept). They may well nap during the day and fall asleep extremely quickly at night.

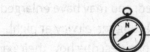

Without consolidated sleep, you will not get the necessary benefits from any sleep you do get.

I often hear from my insomnia patients that they wish they could sleep like their partner, who "falls asleep within seconds, sleeps for at least nine hours a night and also naps for a couple of hours every day". This always worries me, because falling asleep extremely quickly is a sign of sleep deprivation (normal sleepers take around 10–15 minutes to fall asleep). Plus, if you sleep for nine hours a night or more and are still sleepy, then that is a sign that you are not really sleeping properly for those nine hours. In cases like that, I ask to speak to my client's partner, and often refer them to an OSA clinic for assessment!

Warning signs of OSA include snoring and being overweight. When you snore, this indicates a partial restriction in your airway (causing the noise), and if the airway is fully restricted then no air can pass at all. If you are overweight, your throat will be heavier and thicker, and this makes it more likely to press on your airway and close it with gravity. However, snoring is not always weight-related; you may have enlarged tonsils or adenoids impacting the airway at night. Sometimes I hear someone describe how their partner snores noisily but then they will stop for a blissful minute before starting again. Although the partner may think the silence is wonderful, it is in fact an apnoea episode (when their partner is not breathing) – so not such a good thing after all!

OSA is a dangerous condition that needs to be taken seriously – and not only because of the sleep deprivation and daytime fatigue it causes. Each time your body wakes you up from an OSA episode, it does so with a surge in your heart rate and blood pressure. This repeated pressure on your heart every night can lead to hypertension (high blood pressure) and make you more at risk of a heart attack or stroke. If you suspect that you or someone else may have OSA, please speak to a doctor, who will likely recommend an overnight sleep assessment.

OSA needs to be taken seriously – please speak to a doctor, who will likely recommend an overnight sleep assessment.

Treatment for mild OSA may include lifestyle changes, such as losing weight or reducing alcohol consumption, but severe OSA may be treated with continuous positive airway pressure (CPAP) or a mandibular device to force the airway open. CPAP is a mask you wear overnight to force air into your mouth and nose, keeping your airway open. It might not look pretty, but it keeps you alive and gives you a good night's sleep, so it is definitely worth it!

TEETH GRINDING

- Do you wake with a sore jaw?
- Do you have an earache or a headache in the morning?
- Has your dentist told you that you grind your teeth?

If you answered yes to any (or several) of these, you may suffer from **teeth grinding** or bruxism.

Teeth grinding is a condition that causes you to clench or move your top and bottom teeth against each other during your sleep. This can result in jaw pain the next day, as your muscles have been used repeatedly in the night. It can also cause damage and wear to your teeth, which is why a dentist may be the one to alert you to it. Additionally, teeth grinding can be noisy enough to wake you or your bed partner up, causing sleep disturbance for both of you. Often people don't know that they are grinding their teeth at night unless someone else tells them about it.

Teeth grinding is associated with stress and anxiety, consumption of caffeine or alcohol and is more common in people with OSA. Your dentist may recommend wearing a mouth guard at night to protect your teeth and cushion the grinding, helping your sleep in the process.

PERIODIC LIMB MOVEMENT DISORDER

- Do your legs or arms jerk or move uncontrollably during the night?
- Do you feel excessive daytime sleepiness irrespective of how much sleep you have got at night?

If you answered yes to either (or both) of these questions, you may have **periodic limb movement disorder** (PLMD).

Around 80% of people with Restless Legs Syndrome (RLS), which will be explained overleaf, also have PLMD. In both disorders, symptoms are linked to the dopamine levels in the brain. PLMD is where your legs kick out or your arms flail during your sleep, which may disturb your or a bed partner's sleep. Often the movement is regular and occurs around every 20–40 seconds, especially at the start of the night. The person suffering from PLMD may not notice it happening, and it may be a bed partner who draws their attention to it. Symptoms are often associated with lifestyle factors such as excessive caffeine and stress. If you suspect you may have PLMD, speak to your doctor to discuss treatment options. In order to diagnose PLMD, a polysomnography test may be required.

RESTLESS LEGS SYNDROME (RLS)

- Do your legs feel itchy or ache in the evening or when you are tired?
- Do you have the urge to rub your legs in bed?

If you answered yes to either (or both) of these, you may have **restless legs syndrome** (RLS).

RLS is a crawling or itchy feeling in your legs that can only be temporarily relieved by moving, stretching or rubbing them. These uncomfortable feelings are more likely to happen when you are tired and when your legs are still, such as when you are sitting on the sofa in the evening or lying down in bed, making it very hard to get to sleep.

RLS is more common in middle age, but can happen at any time of life, and women are twice as likely to suffer from it than men.

RLS is often caused by a reduction in dopamine levels in the brain. It is more common in middle age, but can happen at any time of life, and women are twice as likely to suffer from it than men. RLS can be associated with lifestyle factors (such as stress, being overweight, caffeine and smoking), underlying health conditions (such as kidney disease, diabetes, Parkinson's disease, rheumatoid arthritis, an underactive thyroid or fibromyalgia), pregnancy, a lack of iron (or low ferritin levels in the blood) or a lack of folic acid. Some medications, such as antidepressants or antihistamines, can also make symptoms worse.

If you suspect that you have RLS, speak to your doctor, who may recommend lifestyle changes such as reducing caffeine, stopping smoking (if applicable) and increasing exercise levels. They may also look into possible causes and prescribe iron supplements if a ferritin blood test suggests you have an iron deficiency.

NARCOLEPSY

- Do you ever feel weak when laughing or emotional?
- Do you ever fall asleep during the day without expecting to?
- Do you have excessive daytime sleepiness irrespective of how much sleep you have had at night?

If you answered yes to any (or several) of these, you may have **narcolepsy**.

Narcolepsy is a condition where people fall asleep during the daytime without intending to. If you have narcolepsy, you may also feel excessively sleepy during the day. In addition to falling asleep unexpectedly (a sleep attack), you may experience **cataplexy**, which is a temporary muscle weakness often brought on by emotion. You may have experienced suddenly feeling very weak when laughing, surprised or angry. This is known as a cataplectic attack. **Sleep paralysis** is also commonly associated with narcolepsy (see page 68).

Narcolepsy is a condition where people fall asleep during the daytime without intending to. You may also feel excessively sleepy during the day.

In order to diagnose narcolepsy, your doctor will likely refer you for a multiple sleep latency test (MSLT). This looks at how quickly you fall asleep at various times of the day, since people with narcolepsy tend to be able to fall asleep extremely quickly. Also, because narcoleptics go straight into REM sleep (rather than the usual N1 stage), a polysomnography test may also be used to confirm diagnosis. If you are diagnosed with narcolepsy, you may be prescribed stimulant medication.

SLEEP PARALYSIS

- Have you woken from sleep to find that you are paralyzed and cannot move or speak?
- Have you woken up terrified to find a strange figure standing at the foot of your bed?
- Have you ever felt like you have floated up above your bed while sleeping at night?

If you answered yes to any (or several) of these questions, you may have experienced **sleep paralysis**.

Sleep paralysis is a REM disorder, meaning it is a problem with dreaming sleep. In REM sleep your body is paralyzed so that you don't physically act out your dreams. During an episode of sleep paralysis, the part of the brain that is conscious and alert wakes up, but the part that keeps you from moving in your sleep remains switched on, which means that you are awake but can't move a muscle – an extremely frightening experience. Indeed, the level of fear can cause the sufferer to imagine that they see a scary figure at the foot of the bed – often a witch, the grim reaper or even an alien. (Very similar scary experiences of ghostly apparitions in the night have been commonly told all over the world for hundreds of years. Likely sleep paralysis episodes have even been reported in newspapers as alien abductions, where the victim had been "paralyzed by the visitor from space".) Sometimes people with sleep paralysis can even feel like they are being lifted up or hovering over their bed, which is caused by the body's confusion over being unable to properly sense and move itself.

Often the scientific understanding of what is happening can help the person experiencing the episode of sleep paralysis feel calmer and less scared when it happens.

Sleep paralysis is commonly found in people with narcolepsy, although this is not always the case. There is no cure, but often the scientific understanding of what is happening, that it is a sleep/wake discrepancy, can help the person experiencing the episode of sleep paralysis feel calmer and less scared when it happens. They can tell themselves that they are not really seeing whatever it is that is frightening them, that they are not really in danger, but rather that their brain has simply woken up while their body is still asleep.

NIGHT TERRORS

- Do you wake, often within the first hour or two of sleep, screaming or terrified?

If you answered yes, you may have experienced **night terrors**. Night terrors are distinct from nightmares, as they do not occur in REM sleep and do not have a plot. Someone experiencing a nightmare will remember it the next day and will be able to describe it to others, whereas night terrors will be completely forgotten by the next morning. The person experiencing a night terror will sit up in bed screaming, possibly with their eyes open. They will seem to be in a huge amount of distress, and it can be a jarring experience for anyone nearby to witness. In fact, they are not really scared at all, because they are still in deep sleep. Night terrors tend to happen soon after falling asleep (around an hour after sleep onset is common), whereas nightmares tend to happen nearer morning. This is because night terrors occur during deep sleep (N3), whereas nightmares occur during dreaming sleep (REM) or stage R. They are a kind of parasomnia (an unusual behaviour that occurs between sleeping and waking or as the person enters or leaves REM sleep).

If you live with someone who has night terrors, the best thing to do is to simply stay calm and wait for the episode to finish rather than trying to wake them up.

A night terror tends to be much more traumatic for the person witnessing it than for the person experiencing it. If you live with someone who has night terrors, the best thing to do is to simply stay calm and wait for the episode to finish rather than trying to wake them up. Night terrors are very common in children (most grow out of them naturally), but sometimes occur in adults – especially adults who also sleepwalk. They are more common when someone is sleep-deprived, jet lagged, has consumed alcohol or doesn't have a good bedtime routine (see page 81, discussing good bedtime routines). If a person regularly has night terrors, a bed partner can sometimes stop them from happening by deliberately waking the person around 15 minutes before the night terror would usually occur, which disrupts their sleep pattern. If night terrors occur most nights or several times per night, you may want to speak to your doctor to see if something else is causing them, such as OSA (page 58) or RLS (page 64).

SLEEPWALKING

- Has someone told you that you got out of bed during the night, but you had no memory of it the next day?
- Do you sometimes wake up in another room of the house or standing up?

If you answered yes to either (or both) of these questions, you may have experienced **sleepwalking**.

Sleepwalking is another parasomnia and is a disorder of deep sleep (N3). Similar to night terrors, sleepwalking occurs when some parts of your brain wake up while other parts remain asleep. However, unlike night terrors, they are less intense. When someone sleepwalks, they will open their eyes, sit up in bed or get up and do basic things that they would normally do during the day, such as walk around the room or go to the kitchen and open the fridge. The person is not acting out a dream, since they are not in dreaming sleep. When someone is sleepwalking, they will be moving slowly, rather than running around, because they are still in deep sleep.

If you know that you sleepwalk, the best thing to do is to make sure that you are safe from any harm that could occur during an episode.

Similar to night terrors, sleepwalking occurs when some parts of your brain wake up while other parts remain asleep.

Sleepwalking is genetic and tends to run in families. An episode is more likely to occur when the person is stressed, has consumed alcohol or is sleep-deprived. If you know that you sleepwalk, then the best thing to do is to make sure that you are safe from any harm that could occur during an episode. Ensure that bedroom windows are locked and consider installing a stair gate at the top of the stairs so that there is less chance of you falling during a sleepwalking episode.

CIRCADIAN RHYTHM DISORDER

- Do you find it hard to fall asleep until the early hours of the morning, but once you are asleep are able to get 7–9 hours' sleep?
- Do you fall asleep very early in the evening but then wake in the early hours of the morning after a reasonable amount of sleep?
- Do you find that you sometimes get a full night's worth of sleep in the middle of the day?
- Do you feel like you wouldn't have a sleep disorder if the whole world would shift its time zone to match yours?

If you answered yes to any (or several) of these questions, you may have **circadian rhythm disorder** (CRD).

Usually, our circadian rhythm is anchored to make us sleepy at night and alert during the day due to our exposure to sunlight (see page 22). However, some people can have a circadian rhythm that is either set to the wrong time (too early or too late) or is free-running, without an anchor to keep it in place. CRD is commonly found in people who are blind, as they aren't able to get the correct circadian stimulation from the sun via their eyes. Their circadian rhythm can therefore change from day to day. For example, they could feel ready for bed at 10pm on Monday, but then feel tired at 8pm the next day, and then 6pm the day after that ... continuing until they are completely at odds with the rest of the population.

Some people can have a circadian rhythm that is either set to the wrong time (too early or too late) or is free-running, without an anchor to keep it in place.

Sometimes, CRD can be advanced, making the person feel sleepy much earlier than appropriate and also waking them much earlier. This can look like a late insomnia issue (a problem with waking up too early), but it is not, as the person has got sufficient sleep – just at a time shifted earlier than they would want. Similarly, delayed CRD is where the person does not feel sleepy until the early hours of the morning, but then they will get a full night's worth of sleep, waking much later in the day. This can also be misdiagnosed as initial insomnia, where the person struggles to fall asleep. Shift work and jet lag can also cause a kind of CRD.

If you suspect you have CRD, speak to your doctor. Treatment may involve light therapy to move your circadian rhythm, or you may be prescribed melatonin supplements.

BEFORE YOU MAKE ANY CHANGES

At this point you hopefully have a better understanding of your sleep, any potential sleep issues, and what the next steps might be. It goes without saying that, first and foremost, if you feel that you cannot cope during the day or you have any thoughts of taking your own life, then it is vital that you seek help straight away from a medical professional. Do not try to handle your important issue alone. (See page 139 for information on the resources that are available to you.)

If you do not feel in a desperate place right now, but you think you may have a sleep disorder such as those described above, then it is important to speak to your doctor for further assessments before making any changes to your sleep. The advice given later on will simply not be effective if there is a medical cause to your sleeping problem. You may like to write down your sleep issues as identified in this chapter and take these notes with you to your doctor's appointment. You may then be enrolled on an overnight sleep study in a hospital or sleep lab, or you may be referred for more tests.

In addition, if you suspect that your sleeplessness and daytime fatigue are caused by another untreated mental health issue (such as depression, anxiety or post-traumatic stress disorder), then it would also be advisable to consult with your doctor to get help for this first. You may need to get whatever issue it is under control before making any changes to your sleep and routines.

If you have identified that you have a temporary sleeping problem (one that has lasted for fewer than three months), then some basic sleep hygiene measures, as discussed in Chapter 4 (page 81), may be all that is needed to help you improve your sleep. Plus, the relaxation exercises and techniques for managing your anxiety about sleep in Chapter 5 may be helpful if you find that you are starting to worry excessively about your sleep and are becoming increasingly anxious.

If you have a sleeping problem that has been ongoing for three months or more (chronic insomnia), then you should check with your doctor for their treatment advice. They are likely to recommend cognitive behavioural therapy for insomnia (CBT-I), as long as the treatment does not conflict with anything else about which the doctor is concerned. A myriad of research has shown that CBT-I provides long-term improvement for insomnia. It works by helping you to change the unhelpful thoughts and behaviours that are keeping you from sleeping. In the UK, doctors no longer prescribe sleeping pills as the first option to treat insomnia, since you can quickly become dependent on them and they can have serious side effects. That said, sometimes doctors will prescribe a short course of sleeping pills (for up to two weeks) while looking at other treatments, or if other treatment options have not worked.

I am a CBT-I therapist, and this is the principle on which much of the advice in this book is based, but this book is not a CBT-I course. However, the advice in the next two chapters may be helpful to help reduce your symptoms prior to accessing full CBT-I. You can access CBT-I through your doctor via talking therapies, via an online app (such as Sleepio, Sleepful or Sleepstation), and you can also see a private qualified therapist (such as myself) or follow the advice given in a CBT-I self-help workbook. The option that will work best for you will depend on the availability of CBT-I provision in your area, your personality (are you a self-directed person who would be able to follow a workbook or online app, or do you do better with support from an individual therapist along the way?) and your finances (one-to-one therapy is more expensive than buying a book). See the resources chapter at the end for more information on how to access CBT-I and further help, as well as links to global resources where you can find help.

The next two chapters contain some fundamental good sleep hygiene advice and some valuable cognitive techniques to help you worry less about your sleep, to help give you a solid foundation for sleep. They may be sufficient to help improve your sleep so that a stronger intervention (such as CBT-I) may not be necessary, and if it is, you will already have a great sleep foundation to work from.

CHAPTER 4

CHANGES TO HELP YOUR SLEEP

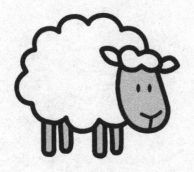

GENERAL GOOD SLEEP HYGIENE

If you are having problems with your sleep, then there are some basic good sleep hygiene principles which can help maximize your chances of sleeping well at night. If your sleep problems are more temporary or less severe, following the advice in this chapter may be enough to solve them. If your sleep problems are more significant, then these are the basics that should be in place before any more intrusive changes are made to your sleep, such as some of the more advanced techniques discussed later or CBT-I.

Before you read about good sleep hygiene, however, remember that everyone is different. There is no perfect template of what to do or what not to do before bed, or what your bedroom should look like. What follows are simply recommendations. If I suggest changing an aspect of your life, bedroom or sleep routine that you currently find pleasant or helpful for your sleep, then don't change it. For example, general good sleep hygiene advice recommends not watching TV or looking at your phone in bed. However, if watching your favourite TV series in bed or playing Sudoku on your phone helps you to relax before you go to sleep, then you don't need to stop doing it.

Once again: *if it isn't broken, don't fix it*. Take from the following advice what you think will work for you and don't worry about the parts you feel don't apply to your situation.

There is no perfect template for what to do or what not to do before bed, or what your bedroom should look like.

DAYTIME CHANGES

There are a number of things you can do during the day which will affect your ability to sleep at night and the kind of sleep that you have. These include exercise, eating the right kinds of food at the right time, exposure to sunlight and dealing with your thoughts and worries during the day instead of at night.

Sunshine

Many people find they have trouble sleeping at night because they do not have a sufficiently robust circadian rhythm. This means that their body and brain do not have a strong sense of the distinction between night and day, or they may be in the wrong time zone. As we have already learned, our internal 24-hour clock is primarily regulated by sunlight intensity during the day. Our brain is pre-programmed to sense light levels (especially blue light frequency) during the daytime and to flag when the maximum lux (or light) of the day is seen, which it then marks as midday. It boosts our alertness during the daylight hours, and produces melatonin to promote sleep when it gets dark.

Many people, however, have problems if they don't physically get outside to see sunlight each day. This can happen if you are stuck in an office and you don't leave to get a break, or if you are working from home and stay indoors. If the only sunshine that you see is on your way home from work at 5 o'clock, then your brain will think that 5pm is in fact midday, and will therefore want you to fall asleep much later than what many would consider a normal bedtime. Similarly, the blue light from LED devices mimics the light frequency your circadian rhythm is looking for. So if you use your phone or laptop at bedtime, you will be making your brain think that it is not time to sleep and that it is still daytime. This causes your brain to suppress melatonin production as it tries to wake you up.

One of the cheapest and easiest things you can do to boost your alertness during the day, and also your ability to sleep well at night, is to simply make sure that you get lots of light exposure during the daytime. Open the curtains wide as soon as you wake up and physically get outside into the sunshine in the

morning. This will help your brain to know that the sun
has risen and that it is daytime.

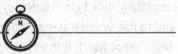

Open the curtains wide as soon as you wake up
and physically get outside into the sunshine in
the morning.

Where possible, go outside for a walk for at least
half an hour at lunchtime, not only to get some
sunlight exposure but also to get a little exercise. For
situations in which you simply cannot get outside
(perhaps you have an unreasonable boss, or it is
raining heavily, or you may be a shift worker), then
think about getting a seasonal affective disorder
(SAD) lightbox. These simulate daylight and are
primarily used to combat the effects of SAD, though
they can also be used to help sleep. Ideally, they
should only be used for a short period of time to
start with as you get used to them (they can cause
dizziness), then gradually build up your use to no
more than an hour a day, some time between 10am
and 1pm depending on your need. They are not
recommended with certain conditions such as bipolar
disorder or epilepsy, so you should check with your
doctor before starting to use an SAD box.

As the day draws to a close, try to dim the lights in the house, as this will help signal to your body that it is getting nearer to bedtime. Make sure that your LED devices (like your phone) are set to night mode, which will automatically reduce the amount of blue light to which you are exposed in the evening. You can even buy special sunglasses which take out the blue light frequency altogether.

Food

When you eat

What you eat during the day not only affects your physical health and sleep, but also your mental health. There is increasing evidence, for example, that our gut is where we create 80% of our happy hormone, serotonin. We know it is important to eat a varied diet full of fresh fruit and vegetables, protein and fibre so that you have all the nutrients your body requires to be healthy, but there are a few other ways in which what – and specifically when – you eat affects your sleep.

As we have already mentioned, your circadian rhythm is primarily regulated by exposure to sunlight. However, it is also influenced (and affected) by when you eat. If you don't regularly eat breakfast soon after waking, then your body is not being given the signals that it is morning and time to start being alert and awake. If you skip lunch or have dinner much too close to bedtime, then once again you are not giving your circadian rhythm the right signals of what time of day it is. Ideally, you should have breakfast, lunch and dinner at regular intervals spaced throughout the day, with breakfast soon after waking, lunchtime in the middle of the day and dinner in the early evening. With jet lag, it is especially important to eat the right meals at the right time of day according to the country that you are currently in. If you eat at the wrong times (either too early or too late), your body will think it is a different time than it really is and adjust your circadian rhythm – and therefore your sleep – accordingly.

Ideally, you should have breakfast, lunch and dinner at regular intervals spaced throughout the day.

In addition to signalling to your body what time it is through eating, your circadian rhythm also controls your body's digestive system and the production of digestive enzymes. Your body is not designed to eat and digest food at night when it should be asleep because your digestive system, in essence, switches off at night. This is why many people who work shifts find they have digestive issues, because our bodies are simply not geared up to deal with food at three in the morning.

Your body gets used to eating at set times of the day. Just imagine how you would feel if you always ate lunch at 12:30pm... As it got closer to midday, your body would begin producing digestive enzymes and your stomach would already be rumbling before you took out your sandwich. It is not a great plan to get into the habit of eating food in the middle of the night, because once you set a pattern, your body would start to actively wake you up with a rumbling tummy because it expected food at that time – in the same way that your tummy expects lunch at 12:30pm if that is when you always eat. Also, eating food during the night will confuse your circadian rhythm into thinking it is already morning and that you are having breakfast at, say, 4am. To avoid waking in the night due to hunger, it is important to make sure that you eat sufficient food during the daytime when your body is supposed to be eating. If you do wake in the night, try to avoid food as well as drinks that are also a "food", such as warm milk. Instead, choose herbal, caffeine-free tea or water.

Food before bed

You may have heard that you shouldn't eat a massive meal right before you go to bed, and this is true. If you eat a lot before going to sleep, your stomach will be bloated; you might have indigestion and falling asleep will be harder. However, if you go to sleep on an empty stomach, then you will be hungry while you're trying to sleep. Evolution has ensured that when humans are hungry, their bodies become anxious and alert enough to make them want to go and forage or hunt for food. Therefore, if you go to bed hungry, rather than preparing for sleep, your body will be telling you to get up and go and find sustenance (nowadays we'd start our search in the fridge rather than embarking on a hunting expedition).

A great idea is to have a small snack of food about an hour before bed. Ideally the food would contain complex carbohydrates (which provide slow-release energy across the night) and dairy (which contains tryptophan – shown to have a small benefit to sleep). A small bowl (smaller than a breakfast portion) of porridge made with milk would be perfect. You could even top it with some fresh kiwifruit, as it has been suggested that kiwi may also aid sleep. If you don't fancy porridge, then a brown bread turkey sandwich or an oat cookie and a glass of milk would also be fantastic. I find it fascinating that we give young children and babies warm milk (and perhaps a cookie) before bed. Without knowing the science behind it, parents naturally do the perfect thing for their young children to help aid their sleep through the night. As we grow up and become adults, however, for some reason we stop doing this for ourselves.

Without knowing the science behind it, parents naturally do the perfect thing for their young children to help aid their sleep through the night.

While we're on the subject of food before bed, if you're wondering whether it's true that cheese causes nightmares, I'm afraid there is no real scientific proof that it does. Cheese is fatty, however, and very fatty food right before bed is more likely to cause indigestion, and so it should be avoided anyway!

Naps

When you are not struggling with sleep at night
If you are *not* having trouble sleeping at night, then a lunchtime power nap can be a fantastic way to boost your general alertness and productivity through the rest of the day. Ideally the power nap should be around 20 minutes (and no longer than 30 minutes). This relatively short duration will ensure that the nap does not significantly affect your sleep drive that night and that you don't find yourself going into the

deepest stage of sleep and wake up feeling groggy. Try not to nap too near to bedtime, and ideally don't nap after 2 o'clock.

When you are struggling with your sleep at night
If you *are* having trouble with your sleep at night, then one of the first things to do is cut out daytime napping altogether. If you can make it through the day without feeling dangerously sleepy, then try your best not to nap. Napping significantly reduces your sleep drive at night, making falling asleep and staying asleep harder. If you must take a nap to help you through the day, then try to make sure that your nap finishes by around 2pm, and ideally make sure that you nap in your bed rather than on the sofa (as we will discuss later in this chapter, it is important to reinforce a positive association between your bed and sleeping, so that you get used to sleeping in your bed).

Napping significantly reduces your sleep drive at night, making falling asleep and staying asleep harder.

Many people have a very short, unintentional "catnap" in the early evening while watching TV, especially when they are struggling to sleep well at night. However, even a tiny 5–10-minute nap will have a detrimental impact on your sleep drive when you get into bed.

Exercise

Getting more exercise during the day is a positive change that you can make to help your sleep. Studies have shown that if you increase the amount of exercise you do during the day, you are likely to have more deep sleep at night. In addition, exercise is also a fantastic stress reliever. When you exercise, you release endorphins, which improve your mood. If you are happier and less stressed, this will help you to feel less anxious at night, which once again makes sleep easier.

There is some evidence to suggest that you should not exercise too close to bedtime, however, as an increased heart rate and temperature make it harder to calm down and fall asleep.

Wind-down time before bed

With small children and babies, parents naturally give them time to wind down before bed. They have a routine that includes, for example, a bath, a last drink of milk, brushing their teeth, putting on pyjamas and reading a story. They may use the same words, songs or scented bubble bath to give further consistency to the sequence of events. Each step of the routine signals to the child that bedtime is on the horizon, which helps their body and brain get ready for sleep.

A parent wouldn't dream of playing tag games with their children five minutes before bed. For the same reason, if we are busy working right up until the moment before we sleep, then our brains will still be in active, alert mode, rather than in relaxing sleep mode. It is very hard to move your mind from the former to the latter at the flick of a switch, without any sort of transition.

Think about a time when you have been in a stressful situation, such as experiencing a moment of road rage perhaps. While the incident is happening, adrenaline will be pumping through your body, your heart will be racing and you will feel very stressed. Do you feel instantly relaxed as soon as the incident, or whatever has caused your stress, has passed? No! Your body and brain need time to calm down. The same thing happens at night. If you are busy and stressed with a work issue and you close your laptop and try to sleep straight away, you will not be able to, because your brain will still be thinking about work and your body will be in a state of anxiety and alertness.

In order to "wind down", try to stop working and looking at electronics around an hour before bed.

In order to "wind down", try to stop working and looking at electronics around an hour before bed. Spend that last hour having a bath, getting your clothes ready for the morning, reading a book and generally preparing for bed. This way there will be a gradual transition from busy work time to sleep time, which will help your body and brain relax and prepare for sleep. Try to keep the lights dim at this time too, to signify to your circadian rhythm that it is nearly time for bed (see page 22).

Caffeine

Caffeine, found in tea, coffee, cola, energy drinks and chocolate, among other foods and drinks, is a very helpful drug to promote alertness, but it can also be very harmful to sleep. Caffeine stops our brain from being able to tell how high our sleep drive is, which makes us feel less tired than we might have otherwise felt, making falling asleep harder.

Have a look at how many caffeinated drinks you are drinking per day, and when you are having them. Caffeine has a half-life of five to seven hours, which means that if you have a cup of coffee within five to seven hours of bedtime, then you will still have approximately half the caffeine still running through your system at that point.

I advise my clients who are struggling with their sleep to switch to decaffeinated drinks after lunchtime. In recent years, decaffeinated tea and coffee has become much, much nicer than it used to be, so it should be easy enough to swap your regular latte for a decaf without feeling too deprived.

If you fall asleep quickly but wake up frequently during the night, you may not think caffeine is a problem for you. However, your sleep drive is still working during the night to help you fall back to sleep again between sleep cycles. Even though your sleep drive may have been high enough for you to fall asleep at the start of the night, despite your after-dinner espresso, three hours later that caffeine is still in your system and it may be stopping your brain from feeling that you have a high enough sleep drive to fall back to sleep again.

Alcohol

Alcohol is a sedative, and so many people find that they start to unconsciously self-medicate for their sleeping problem by increasing the amount of alcohol that they drink before bed, thinking – rightly – that it will help them fall asleep faster. However, in reality, consuming alcohol before bed only results in a poorer quality sleep, especially nearer the morning as it disrupts REM continuity. As we've seen, REM sleep is minimal in the first sleep cycle, but increases as the night goes on. That is why, after quite a few glasses of wine or pints of beer, you might fall asleep (or, more accurately, pass out!) for a couple of hours (for the first part of sleep), but then you would find that you keep waking up for the remainder of the night, as you repeatedly wake up during REM sleep.

If you find that you are drinking more alcohol to help you sleep, or that your sleep is worse when you drink, try cutting back and see if your sleep improves.

Nicotine

Nicotine is a stimulant, and so can cause you to feel too alert to sleep. Having a cigarette if you wake up in the night is therefore not a great idea. Try to avoid smoking near to bedtime, too, if you are struggling to fall asleep.

HOW TO CREATE A GOOD BEDROOM ENVIRONMENT

Your bedroom is where sleep happens, so it is important to make it as conducive to sleep as possible. If your bedroom is not a place where you feel relaxed, safe and comfortable, then falling asleep will be harder. What follows are some ways that you can make sure your bedroom is going to help you fall asleep, rather than be part of the problem.

If your bedroom is not a place where you feel relaxed, safe and comfortable, then falling asleep will be harder.

Calm and clutter-free

If your bedroom is calm and free from clutter, then you will likely feel more relaxed as you lay in bed before falling asleep. If you have piles of unfolded laundry or paperwork lying around, then you might lie in bed and, instead of sleeping, feel like you should be tidying it up. Also, the more mess there is, the more thoughts it will provoke, and before you know it your mind will be racing about something. If your bedroom needs painting or there are picture frames on the floor that you haven't got around to hanging on the wall, then as you are lying in bed your brain will be reminding you of these to-dos instead of allowing you to switch off and sleep. This is one of the reasons that hotel rooms are so minimalistic.

Have an honest look at your bedroom and ask yourself: is it calm and clutter-free? Have you finished those small DIY projects to make your bedroom just as you want it? Do you feel relaxed in your bedroom? If the answer is no to any of these questions, see if there is something you can do to improve your bedroom.

Your bed, mattress and bedding

Your bed is where you physically spend up to a third of your life. You spend more time in your bed than you do in your car or on your sofa. As such, it is really important that your bed is comfortable. If it isn't, then you will struggle to drift off to sleep – especially when you are repeatedly reminded of backaches or even rogue bed-springs sticking into your back!

You spend more time in your bed than you do in your car or on your sofa.

The National Bed Federation (NBF) suggests replacing your mattress approximately every seven years. (Think of it as the seven-year itch!) You should also regularly evaluate the condition of your mattress for signs of obvious wear and tear. A mattress has a natural (finite!) lifespan, and once it starts to feel lumpy or saggy, or you can hear the bedsprings squeak, that is a good indication that your mattress is not supporting you as it should. Your shoulders and hips should sink into the mattress, with your back supported, so that your spine itself stays neutral, instead of being curved. If your mattress is too soft or too firm, then you will wake up during the night as you try to get comfortable.

There are other signs that you might need to replace your mattress. If your bed partner is starting to wake you up as they toss and turn in the bed, this could mean that your mattress has lost some of its support and is not cushioning the movements. Also, if you have put on a significant amount of weight, have become pregnant, or have a new bed partner sharing your bed, then your old mattress may not be sufficient to support this increased weight. You might want to look for a firmer or more supportive mattress. This is why we need to regularly monitor children's mattresses as they grow, for signs that their existing mattress may not be supporting them as they get bigger.

Don't forget to keep your mattress and bedding clean. A mattress protector that can be removed and washed is a great idea, since you can lose around 200ml of fluid through sweat each night (during menopausal night sweats, this figure is even higher). If you don't have a mattress protector, this sweat will go straight into the mattress itself, and you can't put your mattress in the washing machine.

The dead skin cells we lose at night can also be a problem, since asthma-triggering dust mites feed on them and love to live in our mattresses, pillows and duvets. Wash your sheets in a 60-degree wash at least once per week to kill any dust mites, and don't forget to regularly wash duvets and pillows too. By doing this, you also benefit from that wonderful "freshly washed bedding" feeling as you get into bed at night.

It might sound odd, but there is some evidence to suggest that having a separate duvet to your bed partner might also be helpful. Two single duvets in the bed mean that each of you can choose the tog (thickness of the duvet) that suits your needs. Also, when one of you moves, you won't be taking the duvet with you – leaving the other person to sleep more peacefully. In fact, you could go so far as to have separate beds, or even separate bedrooms. When people age and their children leave home, many couples find that they sleep better in separate bedrooms. While some people benefit from the comfort and security of sleeping with a bed partner, it can mean putting up with the other's snoring or restless sleep.

Take the clock out of your bedroom
Do you have a clock in your bedroom that you can see from your bed? If so, it might be a good idea to ditch it, as it can actually exacerbate sleeping problems.

When you are lying in bed trying to get to sleep, or you wake up in the night and look at the clock to check the time, your brain starts to do mental calculations. You might be counting down how much sleep you will be able to get before you need to get up, or contemplating if it is even worth your trying to go back to sleep if you have woken up too early. These mental sleep calculations only serve to stress you more – and, of course, stress is the enemy of sleep. Just because you can't see a clock from your bed doesn't mean you can't check the time. If you have your phone right next to your bed, you will be tempted to reach over and check what time it is.

This temptation can even cause you to wake up properly when you might otherwise have gone back to sleep blissfully unaware of the time. The best thing to do is to not have any clocks visible from your bed and to set an alarm for the morning – facing away from you. If your alarm hasn't gone off yet, then it is still not morning and you can try to go back to sleep. If you do keep your mobile phone in your bedroom, don't have it near enough that you can check it from the bed.

Essential oils
There is some evidence from scientific studies that essential oils, especially lavender, can help you sleep. You could try using a diffuser in the room to fill your bedroom with relaxing fragrances at bedtime, or sprinkle a couple of drops of the essential oil onto your pillow. There are also plenty of pillow sprays on the market you could try. Don't use essential oils when pregnant or in children's rooms, however, and certainly don't use a smell that you don't find pleasant!

Only use your bedroom for sleep (and sex)
If you use your bedroom for activities other than sleep and sex, then it follows that your brain will be thinking about those other things while you are in

bed trying to sleep. For example, if you send work emails from your bed or there is a desk in your room, then while you're trying to get to sleep you'll end up thinking about all the work you still have to do. Similarly, if you have an exercise bike in your bedroom, you might end up feeling guilty about how little exercise you did that day. Your brain will be telling you that instead of sleeping, you should get up and work or do some exercise.

Of course, not everyone has the luxury of having a separate office or exercise room in their house. Therefore, it's important to make a distinction between when you are working or exercising in your bedroom and when you are sleeping. If you have a desk in your bedroom, make sure your work papers and laptop are put away at night. If you have an exercise bike, perhaps put a decorative blanket over it so that you can't see it from your bed. And ideally avoid checking work emails or working on your laptop in bed – designate this space for sleep and sex only.

Ideally avoid checking work emails or working on your laptop in bed – designate this space for sleep and sex only.

Cool and dark bedroom

Try to keep your bedroom cool overnight. As we fall asleep, our body temperature naturally drops. If your bedroom is kept too hot, or your bedcovers are too thick, your body will find it hard to cool down and you will struggle to fall asleep. (That is why it's so difficult to sleep during a heat wave!) Ideally, turn the heating down in your bedroom overnight, open a window and have a lower-tog duvet in the summer than in the winter.

Having a dark bedroom is an obvious way to help you sleep that sometimes gets overlooked. If your curtains let through lots of light, then you will struggle to sleep in the summer when the daylight hours are longer. Even with your eyes closed you can still sense light through your eyelids (try it now!), so when you are trying to fall asleep you might still be disturbed, by car headlights moving through your curtains for example. Again, there's a reason hotel bedrooms often have thick blackout curtains. If your curtains are too sheer, consider replacing them with thicker ones or, even better, installing a blackout blind.

Banish your phone from the bedroom

As we have already touched on, phones and tablets give out blue light, which stimulates our brains to think that it is daytime, making our circadian rhythm suppress melatonin production. In addition to the unhelpful light stimulation from these devices (which you can minimize by activating the night-mode setting), you will also be mentally stimulated by looking at them. You might have intended to go to sleep at 10:30pm, but, before you know it, you find you have been scrolling through social media feeds for an hour. You may even see an upsetting text from a friend or an email from your boss, both of which will cause your mind to start racing. Also, if your phone is next to you in the bed, then you will be motivated to check it if you wake up in the night, which will make you wake up even more.

You don't need to do everything mentioned in this chapter. Simply look at areas where you think you might be able to make some meaningful changes.

Hopefully, this chapter has given you a wide variety of ideas for how you might be able to make some simple daytime changes that will be beneficial for your sleep, in addition to highlighting general good sleep hygiene. You don't need to do everything mentioned here, but simply look at areas where you think you might be able to make some meaningful changes. For many short-term sleeping problems, a few simple tweaks may be enough to solve your sleeping issue. However, for many longer-term insomnias, you may find that your thoughts and anxieties about sleep have become too significant, and that you need to address some of these negative thoughts and anxieties about sleep in order to make improvements. The next chapter will address some ways that you can manage those nighttime and daytime worries, plus give you some practical techniques that you can use to help you relax at bedtime.

CHAPTER 5

STARTING TO ADDRESS YOUR SLEEPING PROBLEMS

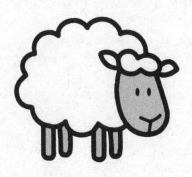

Having ensured that you have good basic sleep hygiene, you may find that your sleep is already starting to improve and, in less severe or short-term cases of insomnia, that those changes are enough to fix the issue. If not, or if you have longer-term chronic insomnia, then don't worry – this chapter builds upon the good sleep hygiene principles you should now have in place and lays out the next set of techniques to start addressing your sleeping problems.

SLEEP DIARY

Now that we are about to discuss some more advanced approaches to fixing your ongoing sleeping problem, this is a good point to introduce the sleep diary. A sleep diary is the most fundamental part of fixing your sleeping problem. By recording each morning how your sleep was the night before, you can develop a more accurate record of your sleep and also spot patterns that may be developing. For example, you may find that your sleep is always worse on a Sunday night, or that you always wake early on a Tuesday when the bins are collected. While you are sleeping poorly it is a good idea to keep a sleep diary every single day for at least two weeks before starting to make changes so that you have a good baseline to which you can compare your improved sleep. You can see how your sleep changes as you use some of the advice suggested in this book. Also, a sleep diary is a useful record to have to show your doctor or CBT-I specialist if you decide to seek professional help for your sleeping issue.

A sleep diary provides a more objective record of what your sleep is like during the course of a week, rather than an emotive look back. For example, you might have one very bad night's sleep and think, *I've not had a good night's sleep for weeks*, but with a sleep diary you can refer back and see that you actually had four good nights in the past seven. Knowing all the facts can help you feel calmer and more in control of your sleep issue. Then, with a regular record, you can start to track your sleep over time, make changes and monitor improvements.

A sleep diary is the most fundamental part of fixing your sleeping problem.

There are several online sleep diaries that you could use to track your sleep, or you can use the template overleaf. Try to record the general impressions of your sleep, rather than looking for accuracy. In other words, don't start to watch the clock, as that will only make things worse. For example, record that you got into bed at about 10pm, and it took you around 30 minutes to fall asleep – not that you got into bed at 10:03pm and took 36 minutes to fall asleep... Also, please do not use a sleep tracker to complete the diary. Instead, write down what *you* thought the timings were and how *you* felt you slept. That is far more important and useful than how your sleep tracker thought you slept, as we discussed earlier (see page 36).

Please do not use a sleep tracker to complete the diary. Instead, write down what *you* thought the timings were and how *you* felt you slept.

Over the page is a suggested structure for your diary and an example of how it might be filled out.

Example sleep diary

Today's date		1st March
Thinking about yesterday		
Q1	Did you take a nap? (Yes/No)	Yes
Q2	If so, how long was the nap?	2 hours
Q3	Did you do any exercise? (Yes/No)	No
Thinking about last night		
Q4	Did you take any sleeping aids to help you sleep? (Yes/No) If so, what and how much?	No
Q5	What time did you get into bed?	10pm
Q6	How long did you take to fall asleep?	90 minutes
Q7	How many times did you wake during the night?	1
Q8	How long in total did you spend awake during the night (after you first fell asleep and before you woke for the last time)?	30 minutes
Thinking about this morning		
Q9	What time did you wake up for the very last time?	5am
Q10	When did you physically get up and out of bed this morning?	8am
Q11	How long did you sleep for in total last night? (TST)	5 hours
Q12	How long did you spend in bed last night? (TIB) (The time between the answers to Q4 and Q11)	10 hours (10pm to 8am)
Q13	How refreshed do you feel, where 1 is not refreshed at all and 5 is extremely refreshed?	2
Q14	How satisfied with your sleep do you feel, where 1 is not satisfied at all and 5 is extremely satisfied?	2
Notes about last night's sleep		
I had a terrible night. I went to bed early but took ages to fall asleep. I woke up at 5am and stayed in bed trying to go back to sleep until 8am. I only got about 5 hours' sleep overall and feel horrible.		

Blank sleep diary template for you to fill in

Today's date		
Thinking about yesterday		
Q1	Did you take a nap? (Yes/No)	
Q2	If so, how long was the nap?	
Q3	Did you do any exercise? (Yes/No)	
Thinking about last night		
Q4	Did you take any sleeping aids to help you sleep? (Yes/No) If so, what and how much?	
Q5	What time did you go into bed?	
Q6	How long did you take to fall asleep?	
Q7	How many times did you wake during the night?	
Q8	How long in total did you spend awake during the night (after you first fell asleep and before you woke for the last time)?	
Thinking about this morning		
Q9	What time did you wake up for the very last time?	
Q10	When did you physically get up and out of bed this morning?	
Q11	How long did you sleep for in total last night? (TST)	
Q12	How long did you spend in bed last night? (TIB) This is how long it was between Q4 and Q11	
Q13	How refreshed do you feel, where 1 is not refreshed at all and 5 is extremely refreshed?	
Q14	How satisfied with your sleep do you feel, where 1 is not satisfied at all and 5 is extremely satisfied?	
Notes about last night's sleep		

As you can see from the example, the sleep diary shows someone who went to bed at 10pm, but who took 90 minutes to fall asleep. They woke up in the night for half an hour but went back to sleep again. They woke up at 5am and tried to go back to sleep until 8am, when they got up. Even though they only got five hours' sleep, they had had a nap of two hours earlier in the day. This means that in the 24-hour period they had actually had seven hours' sleep in total.

ACCEPTANCE

It is important to remember that everyone has nights when they don't get enough sleep. Sometimes the sleep disturbance will be something temporary and outside of your control, such as a sick child needing your attention during the night, or you may be going through a difficult time in your life with a relationship breakdown. As we have already explained, even the best sleepers in the world struggle to sleep well in the midst of a crisis. Most of the time, once the temporary problem stopping you from sleeping improves (e.g. your child gets better) or the longer-term stressful issue starts to lessen (e.g. your relationship issues resolve), your sleeping will naturally improve and go back to normal.

Even the best sleepers in the world struggle to sleep well in the midst of a crisis.

As we have discussed, however, if you start to overly focus on your sleeping problem, and become more anxious about it, then what should have been a short-term issue can persist long beyond the initial cause.

One of the most important things to remember is that a short period of poor sleep is not going to have a significant long-term impact on your health and wellbeing – otherwise every new parent on the planet would be doomed! You will likely have some temporary impairment to your daytime functioning the day after a very poor night's sleep (slower decision-making, etc.), but once your sleep improves again, you will recover from this short-term, temporary sleep loss.

I passionately believe that getting the right amount of sleep is important for maintaining a healthy and happy lifestyle, but worrying excessively about the potential negative health consequences of not getting enough sleep will only make it more likely that the temporary sleeplessness develops into a longer-term issue.

Try to accept that having the occasional bout of bad sleep is completely normal and concentrate on the benefits of improving your sleep, rather than any damage you may be doing by not sleeping well.

Tips for dealing with temporary sleeplessness
What should you do the day after a bad night's sleep? When you have a short period of poor sleep for some reason, there are some things you can do to try to cope during the day and prevent the sleeping difficulty from perpetuating itself.

- Get up at your usual wake time, rather than cancelling your morning plans to have a long lie-in.
- Continue with your daytime plans as usual. Keeping busy will distract you from ruminating on your lack of sleep the night before and show you that you can survive and function on less sleep than you thought (in the short term at least).
- Get as much light exposure as possible during the day. Sunshine will help set your circadian rhythm and also improve your mood.
- You may want to drink a little more tea or coffee (especially in the morning) to perk you up during the day, since caffeine stops our brains from being able to accurately tell how full our sleep drive is. However, as caffeine has a five to seven-hour half-life, make sure you stop ingesting it from around lunchtime.

- If needed, take a power nap of around 20 minutes after lunch. This will give you a boost for the afternoon without disrupting that night's sleep too much.
- Reduce (or avoid) alcohol consumption in the evening. It might help you to fall asleep quickly, but the alcohol will disrupt your sleep later in the night.
- Go to bed at your usual bedtime, rather than going to bed much earlier in an effort to "catch up" on lost sleep.
- In addition, look at the reasons for your sleeping problem, such as relationship worries or job stress. See what practical steps you can take to reduce the root cause of the worries and anxieties affecting your sleep.

Of course, please don't drive or operate any potentially dangerous machinery if you are feeling very tired – it is imperative that you don't put yourself or others at risk.

HABITS AND THOUGHT PROCESSES TO AVOID/ UNLEARN

Thinking about sleep all the time

When you are struggling with sleeplessness, it's hard to think about anything else. You might find yourself noticing how tired you are throughout the day or wondering how your lack of sleep is affecting your ability to work.

The more you are worried about something, the more you pay attention to things related to it during the day. For example, a couple having fertility issues might find they start to see babies and pregnant women everywhere. The same happens with sleeplessness. When you have not slept well, you will notice the bags under your eyes and that pain in your shoulder and blame them on your bad night's sleep. When you drop a cup, you will immediately put it down to the fact that you are so tired. If you had slept well, however, you would see the same bags under your eyes and simply accept that you're not looking your best that day. You might notice the shoulder pain but instead wonder if you'd slept in a funny position the night before. After dropping the cup, you would just think: *Oops!* When you start to attribute normal daytime annoyances *directly* to your sleep, it fuels the notion that your sleep is causing all your problems, which in turn increases your need to fix your sleep and to focus on trying to sleep better.

When you start to attribute normal daytime annoyances *directly* to your sleep, it fuels the notion that your sleep is causing all your problems.

The more you worry about your sleep, the more you will think it has affected your ability to function well during the day. These thoughts also occur at night as you are trying to sleep. You might be lying in bed and start to think, *If I don't fall asleep soon, then I won't be able to go to my friend's BBQ tomorrow because I will be too tired.*

These negative automatic thoughts (or NATs) you have about your sleeping problem go unnoticed and unchecked and become part of your internal rhetoric. Just like the insect, NATs buzz around your head making you feel hopeless and out of control and you can't get rid of them. However, NATs are not facts. They are just thoughts which affect your emotions. When you react to them as if they were true, they shape your mood and seem to confirm your fears that your sleep is a huge problem affecting every aspect of your life.

Negative automatic thoughts are not facts. They are just thoughts that affect your emotions.

In order to stop these negative automatic thoughts, it is a good idea to try to note down any you have about your sleep and sleeplessness in a NAT thought record. First, write down the negative thought, then how that thought makes you feel. Next, consider the truth and accuracy of the thought you had. Think about how else you could explain your feeling; look at the facts rather than your fears. It is important to think about how realistic or truthful your thought is, rather than simply telling yourself to stop worrying or to stop being silly.

Once you have an alternative, more realistic and/or factual thought, the NATs should start to lose their power. You will be able to see the NAT for what it is: a thought, not a fact. Reassessing the thoughts for accuracy can help you feel more in control and less emotionally affected.

The more you stop and notice these NATs, the more you will start to automatically think about the accurate version of them, which is far less worrying than the initial emotive thought. When you don't make an effort to notice these NATs, they will continue to be part of your internal narrative and shape your negative emotions without you even realizing – increasing your underlying stress and anxiety levels.

Copying the example opposite, try noticing your own NATs over the next week and see how many you can reassess for accuracy.

An example NAT Thought Record

My Negative Automatic Thought	Emotional response	Alternative thought (more realistic/factual)	Re-rate your emotional response
I can't function because I am so sleepy.	I feel preoccupied with my lack of sleep and I feel sad.	Perhaps I am just bored (it is a boring meeting), or hungry (haven't eaten for four hours)?	I feel more able to function and more in control, and less sad.
I will never fall asleep tonight.	I feel desperate and extremely anxious.	In the last week the minimum sleep I got was four hours and I averaged five hours' sleep per night, so I am likely to get at least four hours of sleep tonight and probably five.	I feel relieved and more in control. I feel less anxious.
I have a headache because I didn't sleep well last night.	This makes me feel worried about my health.	Perhaps I am thirsty or coming down with a cold?	I feel less anxious and more in control of my feelings.
Everyone else is sleeping except for me.	I feel jealous of other people and very alone.	I know that insomnia is very common, and even the best sleepers have the odd night when they can't sleep.	I feel more normal and less alone.

Spending longer in bed

One of the most common things people start to do when they are struggling to sleep is spend longer in bed trying to catch up on lost sleep. This does seem, on the surface, to be a good idea. If you didn't sleep well last night, then surely you should go to bed early tonight or have a lie-in tomorrow, no? Or perhaps have a nap to get some extra sleep? Unfortunately, all that really happens is that you start to spend longer and longer in bed *not* sleeping.

Has a smell or a taste ever made you remember an event or person from your past? For example, you might smell gasoline and in your mind you are taken back to the happy memory of your father tinkering with his car. You have associated the smell of gasoline with happy times, so that smell makes you happy. This is a positive association.

However, you can also have negative associations. The more time you spend in your bed not sleeping, the more your bed becomes *associated* with not sleeping. When you are lying in bed at night, you probably aren't thinking, *I can't sleep but that doesn't matter. I am happy and relaxed in my bed.* Instead, you're lying there feeling frustrated and annoyed, probably calculating how long you have been trying to fall asleep and how much longer you have left before you have to get up in the morning. Your bed has become a place of anxiety which you associate with not sleeping. This negative association might be so strong that, while you might be feeling very sleepy and even doze off on your sofa, as soon as you get into your bedroom and lie down in your bed, you feel wide awake again. Those feelings of frustration and anxiety pop straight back into your head because of the negative association you have with your bed. Sometimes people even find they sleep better in a spare room, or on holiday or in a hotel room, because those beds have no negative associations.

Trying to accommodate differences between your sleep and your partner's sleep

If you only need seven hours per night, whilst your partner needs nine, neither of you will be happy getting eight hours of sleep per night. I know that it is natural to want to go to bed at the same time as your partner and get up together, but if your sleep needs are different then it is better to go to bed separately, or have different wake times. You can always go to bed early for "snuggle time", and then the partner who needs less sleep can go back downstairs for an hour or two before going to bed when they are ready.

If you only need seven hours per night, whilst your partner needs nine, neither of you will be happy getting eight hours of sleep per night.

COGNITIVE EXERCISES

In addition to dealing with your NATs, here are a number of other cognitive exercises that you can use to help your mind be less active at night as you are trying to sleep:

Expressive writing

If you are too busy during the day to find time to think about important things that are on your mind, then you might find your sleep is disrupted by intrusive thoughts as you try to fall asleep, or you might wake from sleep in the early hours with your mind racing. Make some time (about 15 minutes) to sit down and write about what's going on in your life, anything that's worrying you or causing you stress. Get a journal or just a piece of paper and simply brain dump – it doesn't matter what it is, just write about it. Such expressive writing helps your brain to process your thoughts and emotions, so if you do this ideally a couple of hours before bed, it should stop your brain going through a similar process while you're trying to sleep, or even during sleep itself.

Get a journal or just a piece of paper and simply brain dump – it doesn't matter what it is, just write about it.

Plan tomorrow

If you find yourself worrying about all the things you need to do tomorrow while you are lying in bed, then you might like to deliberately make time to plan your next day's agenda earlier in the day. This might give you focus and make you feel less anxious about the next day, safe in the knowledge that you're fully prepared.

If you note down what is on your mind there and then, then you can let it go and relax, knowing that the reminder will be waiting for you when you wake up in the morning.

Keep a notepad by the bed

Having a notepad and pen within easy reach of the bed is a great idea if you regularly find yourself having niggling thoughts or reminders that pop into your head as you are trying to sleep. For example, if you suddenly remember that you need to book the car in for a service, or that you have to send your grandma a birthday card, then unless you do something about these thoughts, they will continue to go round and round your head, keeping you awake in the process. If you note down what is on your mind there and then, however, then you can let it go and relax, knowing that the reminder will be waiting for you when you wake up in the morning.

Also, don't be tempted to note things down digitally on your phone, as you may get distracted by emails or text messages, and the exposure to blue light will only cause you to feel more awake (see page 83).

Relaxation exercises

Generally speaking, the more anxious you are at night, the harder it will be to sleep. It follows, therefore, that anything that relaxes you will help with your sleep. This could be a body massage during the day, practising mindfulness, or taking a yoga or Pilates class. Perhaps some relaxing essential oils might help you feel calmer. Many people find sleep stories or listening to music in bed calming. There is no exhaustive list of relaxing activities, as this is wholly subjective and personal to each individual. Most of the aforementioned techniques are not specifically recommended as part of the CBT-I approach to curing chronic insomnia; they are just examples of activities that may help you relax, which in turn will help you overcome your temporary sleeplessness.

NAVIGATING SLEEPLESSNESS | 125

If you do something to help you relax, try to do it
purely with that aim in mind.

In the next pages are a number of different exercises
that I recommend for relaxation and therefore better
sleep. It is important to note, however, that anything
you do with the deliberate intention of helping you
fall asleep quicker or to get better-quality sleep will
eventually become associated with poor sleep and
result in the opposite of what you want.

If you do something to help you relax, try to do it
purely with that aim in mind. If you are relaxed, then
you are more likely to sleep, but, more importantly,
you are not spending time in your bed feeling
frustrated and anxious.

PROGRESSIVE MUSCLE RELAXATION

This technique is designed not only to relax your body, but also to give your mind something to focus on instead of being free to wander and possibly start worrying. You can find guided progressive muscle relaxation exercises on YouTube or within relaxation apps such as Headspace or Calm. However, you can easily learn how to do this technique on your own by reading the instructions below and, in many ways, I find that this is even better than relying on a recording. After all, when you are listening to a guided meditation via headphones, you cannot stop the recording if you fall asleep! If you do fall asleep halfway through the relaxation exercise, the voice may well wake you back up again with the next relaxation command. If you can try to do this progressive muscle relaxation exercise by yourself (in your own mind), then you will hopefully finish mid-way – or as soon as you fall asleep! Also, if you are focusing on how to do the exercise, then your mind is also less likely wander, because you are too busy concentrating on the task at hand.

How to do it:
You can do this progressive muscle relaxation exercise any time of day when you would like to relax, but especially as you are trying to fall asleep, either at the

start of the night or when you want to get back to sleep after waking during the night. It can be done sitting in a chair or lying down and should take approximately ten minutes. I recommend that you read through the script below a couple of times before you try to do it on your own at night. Remember that you do not have to stick to this method exactly; what follows is a general guide for how to progressively move up your body, tensing and relaxing different muscle groups as you go.

- Lie down in your bed (or sit in a chair if you prefer) and gently close your eyes.
- Begin by concentrating on your toes. Become aware of their presence and pay attention to how they feel. Focus all your attention on them. Consciously tense them, as if grabbing sand between each one. Pay attention to the feeling of them being tense and hold that feeling for a few seconds. Slowly uncurl your toes and feel them relax.

Remember that you do not have to stick to this method exactly. Read through the script a couple of times then try to do it on your own at night.

- Next concentrate on your ankles. Focus all your attention on them. Imagine them becoming tense. Pay attention to the tension and how heavy they feel. Hold on to that sensation for a few seconds before mentally relaxing your ankles. Imagine that your feet and ankles are heavier and sinking deeper down into the mattress.

- Now think about your calf muscles. Pay attention to how they feel. Do they feel heavy or tense? Consciously increase the tension in your calves and hold that tension for a few moments. Then release the tension and feel them relax and sink down into the mattress, heavier than before.

- Repeat this process with your knees, upper legs, thighs, pelvis and buttocks.

This technique is designed not only to relax your body, but also to give your mind something to focus on instead of being free to wander and possibly start worrying.

- Next concentrate on your chest and your breathing. Pay attention to the rhythm of your breathing for a few moments. Consciously take a deep breath in, filling your lungs to the bottom of your chest, and hold it for a few seconds, tensing your whole chest. Then breathe out as if you were slowly blowing up a balloon, fully emptying your lungs. Deepen your breathing slightly and feel your whole chest sink down into the mattress.

- Now pay attention to your fingers and palms. Focus on each finger and the weight of your palms. Slowly tense your fingers as if gripping a piece of cloth in your hands and hold for a few moments. Then gently relax your fingers and feel each hand get heavier and sink into the mattress.

- Move up to your lower arms. Focus on the sensation of how heavy they feel. Consciously tense and then relax them before feeling them sink down into the mattress.

- Repeat with your upper arms and biceps.

- Now pay attention to your shoulders. We hold a great deal of tension and stress in this part of the body. Can you feel any tension there? Intentionally pull them tight and hold the tension for a few seconds, before slowly relaxing them and feeling the tension slide away.

- Next move to your neck. Pay attention to its weight. Pull your neck muscles tense and hold for a few seconds. Then let the muscles relax and sink down into the mattress.

- Now consider your head and skull. Think about your brain inside guiding everything that you do. Feel the weight of your head. Intentionally tense your head muscles and hold on to that tension for a few moments before relaxing. Feel your whole head become heavier and sink deeper into your pillow.

- Next, concentrate on your mouth and jaw. We tend to hold a great deal of tension in our jaw muscles as well. Can you feel any stress or tightness here? Intentionally clench your jaw and hold for a few seconds. Then slowly relax and unclench your jaw muscles. Feel your mouth and jaw become relaxed and heavier.

- Now think about your eyes. Can you feel any tension in your eyes? Gently tighten your eyelids and keep them shut for a few moments before releasing. Feel any remaining tension slide off your eyes and off your face.

- Next, concentrate on your face and cheeks. Focus on tensing them for a few moments and then consciously let them relax.

- Lastly, mentally scan your whole body for any remaining tension. If you find somewhere that still feels tense, consciously relax that part of your body and then let it become heavier and sink into the mattress.

VISUAL IMAGERY

This technique is about creating your "happy place" – somewhere you can mentally travel to when you are feeling stressed or anxious, or trying to fall asleep.

First, you need to choose the setting. It could be a beach, a forest, a clearing by a lake, or any place where you would enjoy sitting and relaxing. Once you have thought of a place you would like to be, close your eyes and start to imagine what it would look, sound, feel, smell and even taste like.

Say you were to choose a beach. Imagine that you are sitting on the warm sand looking out to sea. Picture the sea. Does the sunlight sparkle and glisten off the crests of the waves? Imagine what the waves sound like as the water hits the shore. Can you imagine the feeling of the sea spray on your face? What does it feel like? What does it taste like? Can you feel the sea breeze on your face? What does the sea smell like? What else can you see? Are there any birds high up in the sky? Can you hear them? Are there any ships on the horizon, or any people swimming in the sea? Now feel your hands. Run them across the warm sand and try to pick up a handful. Can you feel the grains of sand run through your open fingers? Do they feel warm and soft? Now really look at the sand in your hands. Imagine the different colours of the individual grains of sand and the size of the grains. Now think about the trees and plants on the beach. Can you see palm trees or grasses? Can you see their leaves moving in the breeze? Can you imagine the individual leaves on the trees or the individual blades of grass? Can you hear the rustling of them moving gently in the breeze?

The image described above is vivid and full of not only visual imagery, but also sounds, textures, smells and tastes. Your own mental image should also be full of detail and employ all of your senses. The more detailed the scenery, the more believable and engaging it will be. The more complex it is, the less mental capacity you'll have to worry or think about anything else.

I would suggest adding detail to your "happy place" at points during the daytime, so that when you come to think of it in bed you are not spending time and effort creating a brand new image – you are remembering one you have already worked on.

When you lie down in bed and close your eyes you should be able to pull straight to mind this wonderfully engaging and descriptive relaxing scenery. Once you have created one scene, there's nothing to stop you creating others, either. The only limit is your imagination.

4-7-8 BREATHING

This is another excellent technique to use when you are stressed or anxious, or when in bed trying to fall asleep.

As we have discussed, when you are stressed or anxious, your fight-or-flight response kicks in. This means that your heart starts beating more quickly and your breathing becomes faster and shallower. Your body does this so that you are able to pump more oxygen around your body, in case your muscles need extra oxygen to help you fight or run away from a physical threat. The 4-7-8 breathing technique is fantastic because it artificially slows your breathing down to a rate that your body usually only associates with extreme calmness.

The 4-7-8 breathing technique is fantastic because it artificially slows your breathing down to a rate that your body usually only associates with extreme calmness.

How to do it:
You can do this breathing exercise at any time of day when you feel yourself getting stressed and breathing too quickly, but especially as you are trying to fall

asleep at the start of the night or after waking up during the night.

- Start by placing your tongue against the roof of your mouth just behind your teeth.
- Breathe in through your nose for a count of four, holding your tongue in place. As you breathe in, try to fill your lungs right to the back and deep down into your chest. (When we are stressed, we tend only to breathe at the very top of our chest. If you deliberately breathe much lower down, filling your whole lungs, this is much more relaxing breathing.)
- Once you have breathed in for a count of four, hold that breath for a count of seven.
- After seven counts, purse your lips as if you are about to blow up a balloon and breathe out slowly but consistently for a count of eight. You can even use a whooshing sound as you breathe out.

The first few times you try this breathing technique, repeat it just a couple of times (4-7-8, 4-7-8) and then slowly build up over time to a maximum of eight repetitions at any one time.

REPEAT THE WORD "THE"

This is a very simple but remarkably effective technique to stop those persistent nagging thoughts that run through your head while you are trying to get to sleep. Simply repeat the word "the" inside your head about every two seconds until the unwanted thought disappears. The reason we use the word "the" is because it has no negative connotations; it is a neutral word.

Saying the word over and over again disrupts the unwanted thought pattern because it is almost impossible to hold two thoughts in your head simultaneously.

Saying the word over and over again disrupts the unwanted thought pattern because it is almost impossible to hold two thoughts in your head simultaneously. If you've ever tried to remember something, like a WiFi password, while someone bombards you with other information, you'll know what I mean!

FURTHER STEPS

Hopefully, by this point, by better understanding sleep in general and your own sleep in particular, improving your sleep hygiene and employing some of the cognitive and relaxation techniques above, you will have helped or may even have completely resolved your sleep issues. You may be empowered to take some steps to put yourself first and to prioritize your own sleep and wellbeing.

However, with chronic insomnia (as already defined on page 54), changes to your bedtime routine and sleep hygiene may not be sufficient to improve your sleep. The fact is that the unhelpful sleep behaviours and worry about your sleeping problem that you have developed over time may be so ingrained that you need specific, targeted strategies to overcome them. This is where CBT-I comes into its own.

If you feel that you may be a candidate for CBT-I, then I would strongly recommend that you seek advice from a CBT-I specialist. Science has proven that CBT-I is highly effective in overcoming chronic insomnia, but it is not without risk, and I would never advise trying it without first discussing it with a medical professional. Details on how to find a qualified CBT-I professional are included on page 142.

WHERE TO FIND HELP AND OTHER RESOURCES

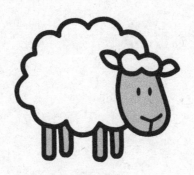

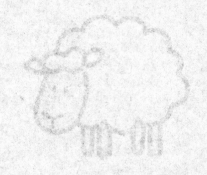

Hopefully you have learned a great deal about sleep and how to navigate sleeplessness in this book. This last section will direct you to further sources of help.

GENERAL MENTAL HEALTH SUPPORT

If your sleeping issue has made it hard for you to cope during the day, there are a number of organizations who can help or signpost you to the right support:

UK

- Heads Together: www.headstogether.org.uk
- Hub of Hope: www.hubofhope.co.uk
- Mental Health Foundation UK: www.mentalhealth.org.uk
- Mind UK: www.mind.org.uk
- Rethink Mental Illness: www.rethink.org
- Samaritans: Helpline: 116 123 E-mail jo@samaritans.org. www.samaritans.org
- Scottish Association for Mental Health (SAMH) (Scotland): www.samh.org.uk
- Shout: www.giveusashout.org, text 85258
- Young Minds: www.youngminds.org.uk

Europe

- Mental Health Europe: www.mhe-sme.org

USA

- HelpGuide: www.helpguide.org
- Mentalhealth.gov: www.mentalhealth.gov
- Mental Health America: www.mhanational.org
- National Alliance on Mental Illness (NAMI):
  www.nami.org
- National Institute of Mental Health:
  www.nimh.nih.gov
- Very Well Mind: www.verywellmind.com

Canada

- Canadian Mental Health Association: www.cmha.ca
- Crisis Service Canada: www.ementalhealth.ca

Australia and New Zealand

- Beyond Blue: www.beyondblue.org.au
- Head to Health: www.headtohealth.gov.au
- Health Direct: www.healthdirect.gov.au
- Mental Health Australia: www.mhaustralia.org
- Mental Health Foundation of New Zealand:
  www.mentalhealth.org.nz

SLEEP ORGANIZATIONS

UK

- British Sleep Society (BSS): www.sleepsociety.org.uk
- The British Snoring and Sleep Apnoea Association: www.britishsnoring.co.uk
- The Sleep Charity: www.thesleepcharity.org.uk

Europe

- European Sleep Research Society (ESRS): www.esrs.eu

USA

- American Academy of Sleep Medicine (AASM): www.aasm.org
- Sleep Research Society (SRS): www.sleepresearchsociety.org

Canada

- Canadian Sleep Society: www.css-scs.ca

Australia and New Zealand

- Sleep Health Foundation: www.sleephealthfoundation.org.au

CBT-I THERAPISTS

Organizations which have lists of qualified experts are:

- The British Association for Behavioural and Cognitive Psychotherapies (BABCP) (UK): www.babcp.com
- British Psychological Society (BPS) (UK): www.bps.org.uk
- Society for Behavioural Sleep Medicine (SBSM) (USA): www.behavioralsleep.org

ONLINE CBT-I

- Sleepful: www.sleepful.me
- Sleepio: www.sleepio.com
- Sleepstation: www.sleepstation.org.uk

RELAXATION AND MINDFULNESS RESOURCES

There are several apps which specialize in relaxation techniques and nighttime sounds/white noise and sleep stories. These can be helpful to help you calm down and be more relaxed at bedtime, which may then help you get to sleep more easily.

- Calm: www.calm.com
- Headspace: www.headspace.com

REFERENCES

Berry, R. B., Quan, S. F., Abreu, A. R., Bibbs, M. L., DelRosso, L., Harding, S. M., et al. (2020). *The AASM Manual for the Scoring of Sleep and Associated Events: Rules, Terminology and Technical Specifications*.

Fultz, N. E., Bonmassar, G., Setsompop, K., Stickgold, R. A., Rosen, B. R., Polimeni, J. R., & Lewis, L. D. (2019). Coupled electrophysiological, hemodynamic, and cerebrospinal fluid oscillations in human sleep. *Science, 366*(6465), 628–631.

Hirshkowitz, M., Whiton, K., Albert, S. M., Alessi, C., Bruni, O., DonCarlos, L., et al. (2015). National Sleep Foundation's sleep time duration recommendations: methodology and results summary. *Sleep Health: Journal of the National Sleep Foundation, 1*(1), 40–43.

Shi, G., Xing, L., Wu, D., Bhattacharyya, B. J., Jones, C. R., McMahon, T., et al. (2019). A Rare Mutation of β1-Adrenergic Receptor Affects Sleep/Wake Behaviors. *Neuron, 103*(6), 1044–1055.

Trump, D. J., & McIver, M. (2004). *Trump: Think Like a Billionaire: Everything You Need to Know About Success, Real Estate, and Life*.

Xiao, Q., Arem, H., Moore, S. C., Hollenbeck, A. R., & Matthews, C. E. (2013). A Large Prospective Investigation of Sleep Duration, Weight Change, and Obesity in the NIH-AARP Diet and Health Study Cohort. *American Journal of Epidemiology, 178*(11), 1600–1610.

Triggerhub.Org is one of the most elite and scientifically proven forms of mental health intervention

Trigger Publishing is the leading independent mental health and wellbeing publisher in the UK and US. Clinical and scientific research conducted by assistant professor Dr Kristin Kosyluk and her highly acclaimed team in the Department of Mental Health Law & Policy at the University of South Florida (USF), as well as complementary research by her peers across the US, has independently verified the power of lived experience as a core component in achieving mental health prosperity. Specifically, the lived experiences contained within our bibliotherapeutic books are intrinsic elements in reducing stigma, making those with poor mental health feel less alone, providing the privacy they need to heal, ensuring they know the essential steps to kick-start their own journeys to recovery, and providing hope and inspiration when they need it most.

Delivered through TriggerHub, our unique online portal and accompanying smartphone app, we make our library of bibliotherapeutic titles and other vital resources accessible to individuals and organizations anywhere, at any time and with complete privacy, a crucial element of recovery. As such, TriggerHub is the primary recommendation across the UK and US for the delivery of lived experiences.

At Trigger Publishing and TriggerHub, we proudly lead the way in making the unseen become seen. We are dedicated to humanizing mental health, breaking stigma and challenging outdated societal values to create real action and impact. Find out more about our world-leading work with lived experience and bibliotherapy via triggerhub.org, or by joining us on:

🐦 @triggerhub_

ⓕ @triggerhub.org

📷 @triggerhub_